THE
RED
WINE
DIET

THE
RED
WINE
DIET

ROGER CORDER

AVERY
a member of Penguin Group (USA) Inc.
New York

AVERY

Published by the Penguin Group
Penguin Group (USA) Inc., 375 Hudson Street, New York, New York 10014, USA · Penguin Group (Canada),
90 Eglinton Avenue East, Suite 700, Toronto, Ontario M4P 2Y3, Canada (a division of Pearson Penguin Canada Inc.) ·
Penguin Books Ltd, 80 Strand, London WC2R 0RL, England · Penguin Ireland, 25 St Stephen's Green, Dublin 2, Ireland
(a division of Penguin Books Ltd) · Penguin Group (Australia), 250 Camberwell Road, Camberwell, Victoria 3124, Australia
(a division of Pearson Australia Group Pty Ltd) · Penguin Books India Pvt Ltd, 11 Community Centre, Panchsheel
Park, New Delhi–110 017, India · Penguin Group (NZ), 67 Apollo Drive, Rosedale, North Shore 0745, Auckland,
New Zealand (a division of Pearson New Zealand Ltd) · Penguin Books (South Africa) (Pty) Ltd, 24 Sturdee Avenue,
Rosebank, Johannesburg 2196, South Africa

Penguin Books Ltd, Registered Offices: 80 Strand, London WC2R 0RL, England

First published in the United Kingdom by Sphere, 2007
First trade paperback edition published in the United States by Avery, 2007

Copyright © 2007 by Roger Corder

Most Avery books are available at special quantity discounts for bulk purchase for sales
promotions, premiums, fund-raising, and educational needs. Special books or book excerpts also
can be created to fit specific needs. For details, write Penguin Group (USA) Inc. Special Markets,
375 Hudson Street, New York, NY 10014.

Library of Congress Cataloging Control Number : 2007932668

ISBN 978-1-58333-290-0

Printed in the United States of America
1   3   5   7   9   10   8   6   4   2

BOOK DESIGN BY TANYA MAIBORODA

To Sue, my epicurean companion

contents

1

YOU are WHAT YOU eat (and DRINK)

WINE DRINKERS GENERALLY are healthier and often live longer than people who don't drink wine on a regular basis. This is not just wishful thinking. I've spent many years researching the health-giving benefits of wine, and I've found that wine drinkers have a lower incidence of heart disease and diabetes, and are also less likely to suffer from dementia in old age than non-wine drinkers. Is this the wine, their diet, or their lifestyle? Well, it's probably a mixture of all three. In *The Red Wine Diet* I examine the importance of these aspects for achieving optimal well-being and I argue the case for daily consumption of red wine as part of a healthy lifestyle. For those who do not want to drink red wine, I suggest some alcohol-free alternative food and drinks that can provide a similar benefit.

My advice is based on studies of the food, wine, and way of life of some of the healthiest, longest-living people in the world. Over the past twenty years, the idea that red wine is good for you has become widely accepted. It was driven to prominence by the belief that wine consumption is at the bottom of what is known as the French paradox—the statistical phenomenon of a relatively low level of heart disease in France despite a high level of consumption of saturated fat.

The solution to the French paradox is more complicated than simply saying that all wine is good for you. But with nutritious food and moderate quantities of the right kinds of red wine, everybody can enjoy good health and all the pleasures of life.

WINE, THE GREAT PROTECTOR

Wine—the fermented juice of grapes—has many components, but which of these are most important for improving well-being? To help you understand how scientists are investigating this topic, I describe the latest research. This comes from my own laboratory, and also from many others in this field who are trying to unravel the precise protective properties of different dietary components. This introduces the topic of dietary polyphenols, a diverse group of several thousand plant chemicals. For many of them we do not yet know the full extent of their actions, and their contribution to overall health and well-being is only just beginning to be understood. These polyphenols come in many forms, but which ones are important?

Healthy blood vessels are the key to keeping your heart, brain, and every other organ in good shape. Healthy blood vessel function may also help prevent cancer. So I have included the findings of research in my lab that focused on identifying the vascular-protective constituents of wine. In a nutshell, we identified procyanidins (sometimes called proanthocyanidins), the most abundant polyphenol in young red wines, as the key health component of wine.

There are a wide number of dietary sources of procyanidins. These plant chemicals are abundant in nature, although modern food processing does much to eliminate them. There may well be more to the saying "An apple a day keeps the doctor away" than has been realized. Cranberries are another rich source of procyanidins. Procyanidins are also the main polyphenols in cocoa and chocolate, which itself has a history of consumption for its health benefits. Procyanidins are just one subgroup of the many thousands of dietary polyphenols. Pomegranates and walnuts contain other types of polyphenols that also have potent positive effects on blood vessels. So if you want to avoid drinking alcohol, there are other ways to increase your daily consumption of vascular-protective polyphenols.

YOUR HEALTH IS IN YOUR HANDS

Health care is big business. From large pharmaceutical companies to chain-store pharmacies, and from the open-heart surgeon to the general practitioner/family physician, enormous sums of money are spent on helping people stay "healthy." However, despite the fantastic progress over the past fifty years, particularly with new medicines and more advanced diagnostic equipment, I can't help thinking these improvements sometimes encourage ill health. Too many complacent consumers expect "a pill for every ill" or are overwhelmed by the suicidal hedonism inherent in the philosophy "you only live once" and treat it as an excuse for habits that will almost certainly take them to an early grave. A different approach might make their one life longer yet no less enjoyable.

Consumers can be their own worst enemies. Studies of the factors that affect food choice have found that in countries with a well-resourced provision of health care, the shopping patterns and eating habits of consumers are influenced less by the need to eat healthily. Researchers think this is due to consumers' expectation that the health care system will be there as a safety net for their wayward habits and excesses. This philosophy is flawed. The chronic conditions of diabetes and heart disease can be avoided. Prevention is better than cure! To illustrate this point, it is widely accepted that costly bypass surgery for coronary heart disease saves many lives. But if a radical change in diet and lifestyle doesn't occur at the same time, then five years after surgery the risk of sudden death is the same as if the operation had not taken place. So the goal of *The Red Wine Diet* is to provide a fresh outlook on how to stay healthy.

Societies with some of the healthiest, longest-lived people—Sardinia, Crete, rural southwest France—often lack state-of-the-art health services and facilities, yet their inhabitants still live to a ripe old age because they take better care of themselves, eat a high percentage of fresh and unprocessed foods, and drink wine every day. Everybody needs to place greater emphasis on keeping themselves healthy as a tactic for greater long-term quality of life with less dependence on medical care. Throughout this book I would like to provoke a greater sense of the need for self-reliance when it comes to our health. Eating nutritious food is an absolutely essential first step.

YOU ARE WHAT YOU EAT

Recent reports indicate that life expectancy in the United States and in parts of Europe is actually decreasing. Much of this alarming new trend is the result of the dramatic increase in obesity. While many think that excess consumption of sugar and saturated fats is the only evil that needs to be eradicated, it is clearly much more complicated than this.

For many people, living life at their ideal healthy weight is a constant struggle. Is this because of the food we eat or the life we lead? Health professionals have been unable to provide a reliable solution to this problem, and the conflicting advice from various government authorities, health organizations, and diet gurus has created a state of confusion. It is even more worrying that diets and dieting are often driven by fashion and fads, without evidence that they guarantee a long-term benefit to health. In *The Red Wine Diet* I discuss some of the key health issues facing us and the contribution poor nutrition makes to these problems.

Weight-loss diets are frequently lacking in essential nutrients and put you at risk of becoming ill rather than glowing with health. Before resolving to diet it is important to be aware of an almost unbelievable fact: many overweight people are suffering from a type of malnutrition and crash diets usually make this worse. If you are wondering how this can be possible, the answer is quite simple. We evolved living off relatively low-calorie food, which meant we had to eat more to obtain enough energy to survive. In doing so we consumed more micronutrients—the vitamins and minerals that our bodies need to keep every cell in a healthy state. Over the past hundred or so years the Western diet has become increasingly rich in calories. So now the number of calories required to live can be obtained from a smaller quantity of food. But this means that micronutrient consumption has decreased.

To compound the problem, over the past twenty to thirty years lifestyles have changed: energy expenditure has been reduced through jobs that are more often sedentary and everyday lives that don't require any exercise. We no longer need to spend day after day searching for food—we can pick up the phone and get pizza delivered to our door. Our calorie needs therefore have become smaller. At the same time, our food is increasingly processed away from its natural state, and many people living on calorie-rich foods are deficient in vitamins and minerals. This has led many adults and children to suffer from a condition known as type B malnutrition. Whether you are overweight or in the healthy range, if your diet is high in fries and pizza but lacks fruits and vegetables, you could be suffering from some degree of malnutrition! Although the health consequences of this type of malnutrition are not comparable to those experienced by the starving populations in sub-Saharan Africa, its impact on long-term well-being is becoming apparent. Obesity is not only linked to increased heart disease but also to cancer. Inadequate consumption of specific vitamins and minerals increases the likelihood of these diseases. So perhaps it is time to think less about your weight and more about what you eat.

Going on a diet is generally taken to mean adopting a regime that restricts intake of food and drink, with the aim of losing weight. But this may mean a reduction in the consumption of important nutrients to the point that harm is done. Most "diets" also exclude alcoholic drinks. Yet medical evidence suggests that regular consumption of alcohol can be part of a healthy lifestyle. This book not only provides nutrition advice that will help you improve your health but also gives guidance on how to make the most of regular wine consumption as part of a sensible pattern of wine drinking. The best diets are for life, not just to recover from Christmas or other periods of feasting. A healthy diet should be complete in every way, so that nothing is lacking and nothing is in excess. This book provides lifestyle and dietary advice that will help achieve this goal and therefore provide the greatest long-term benefit to health. If followed carefully, you should lose weight in the process.

To highlight specific issues for achieving maximum well-being the focus of each chapter is different. But all the topics are interconnected as part of a common goal of living well for good health and a longer life.

LIVING TO BE a HEALTHY centenarian

You may feel that the last thing you want to be is 100 years old and so decrepit that your continued existence is completely dependent on the care of another person. But that is not the life of every nonagenarian or even centenarian. An ever-growing number of studies show that people living active healthy lives, often with a glass or two of wine a day, live the longest. Being active and eating a balanced selection of healthy foods is an absolute necessity. As soon as these good habits wane, general health tends to decline. Dementia and failing eyesight are major worries for many elderly people—both are influenced by diet. Many elderly people become reluctant to eat proper meals, particularly if they are eating alone. Instead they choose high-calorie or ready-made options that are nutritionally inadequate. This is a completely wrong approach. Aging bodies need fewer calories and use vitamins and minerals less efficiently. For optimum good health, calories should be matched to needs, and diet should be varied, with plenty of fruits and vegetables.

Research to discover the secrets of longevity inspires great interest. The motivation is generally driven by the idea that a secret formula can be discovered that will enable us all to live beyond our normal life expectancy. Many investigations focus on healthy populations with a high proportion of centenarians. My own endeavors in this area include investigating the wine people drink in Sardinia, Crete, southwest France, and Georgia (the former Soviet Republic). Our results provide several new insights into the type of wine that is best for long-term health. This research also indicates that the French paradox is not a statistical aberration, but that it reveals a fundamental aspect of diet and health we should spend more time researching.

DRINKING YOUR HEALTH

It is important to recognize what represents healthy wine drinking—and what habits the wine drinker should avoid! Whether all red wines confer the same benefits is another interesting question for wine drinkers. Tests in my lab show that some red wines contain much higher levels of procyanidins (the protective polyphenols that improve blood vessel function) than others. By drinking these wines, maximum benefit can be gained while drinking less. So how do you know which wines to choose? In Chapter 7, I describe some of the most beneficial wines I have found. They have many common features, including vineyard practice, grape variety, and winemaking style, and I provide detailed information on these characteristics so you can seek out other wines with similar properties. All are the perfect accompaniment for food, and that is the best way of gaining the health benefits of drinking wine.

IMPROVING YOUR HEALTH
THROUGH DIET AND LIFESTYLE

Most illnesses are dealt with by medical or surgical interventions that control the symptoms or alter the course of disease. A better approach would be to focus on staying healthy throughout life so that diseases such as cancer become less common. We should also devote more resources to understanding what happens during the aging process so that old age can become a period of maintained vitality rather than a phase in life where the only expectation is declining health.

Increasingly we are recognizing that chronic progressive diseases such as heart disease, diabetes, dementia, and several forms of sight loss have a number of common underlying symptoms. The most important of these appears to be abnormalities in blood vessel and capillary function. Recent research has revealed some surprising findings. For instance, osteoporosis is more common in people with risk factors for heart disease. Is this because a diet and lifestyle that favors heart disease also increases the likelihood of osteoporosis? Or do vascular abnormalities occurring with heart disease also alter bone metabolism in a manner that triggers osteoporosis?

I also discuss dietary factors that influence the risk of cancer. Diets rich in flavonoids (a type of polyphenol) not only reduce the level of heart disease but also reduce the frequency of cancer. This might be because these plant chemicals block the growth of cancerous cells, or it may be that flavonoids, such as those in red wine, act by improving vascular health, which then makes it more difficult for tumors to grow or for cancerous cells to spread.

Being overweight increases the likelihood of a number of health problems. Eating the wrong foods only makes things worse. It is important to follow a diet that helps avoid weight gain but also improves overall health. Fat has been the villain of the food and weight-loss industry for the past twenty or so years, but some fat is good for you. The term *essential fatty acids* refers to fats you need to eat to stay healthy. Fat also aids in the absorption of some vitamins and other nutrients. Diets very low in fat are not the best option if you want to be in tip-top health.

The Red Wine Diet emphasizes the importance of complete nutrition for maximum well-being. Where a balanced diet focuses on the need for a mix of foods for their carbohydrate, fat, and protein content, complete nutrition means consuming a variety of foods to ensure that essential nutrients, vitamins, and minerals are included as part of a balanced diet. I combine some recommendations for good foods to eat with a gentle education about why particular lifestyle and eating habits can be risk factors for illness. Exercise is crucial for providing the right balance between calorie consumption and energy expenditure; exercise will also give you greater energy and a more positive self-image. I believe that a better understanding of how dietary factors affect health will convince you of the importance of making changes. If you feel unable to give up a particular habit immediately, you may well be able to adapt gradually to a healthier diet and lifestyle knowing what the consequences might be if you don't.

I also weigh up the arguments for obtaining complete nutrition from the food you eat rather than relying on vitamin and mineral supplements the efficacy of which has not been proven through clinical trials. Detailed investigations of high-dose vitamin supplements have sometimes found that they do more harm than good. For optimal health the best diets are composed of many different nutritionally important foods that are varied over a cycle of a week or more in order to keep you topped up with all of the essential vitamins and minerals.

As I've mentioned, the Red Wine Diet is a healthy eating plan that does not require you to drink wine or other alcoholic beverages to enjoy its benefits. But as when making any change in diet, avoid foods to which you or your family members may have allergies or other types of sensitivities. If you are pregnant or do not normally drink alcoholic beverages, you should not start drinking wine without first discussing it with your doctor. If you have a history of liver disease or health problems associated with alcohol consumption, then you should avoid wine altogether.

RECIPES FOR HEALTH

My recipes are easy to make and geared to providing complete nutrition. They form the basis of *The Red Wine Diet*, which is a Mediterranean-style diet that incorporates daily consumption of red wine as part of a healthy lifestyle. For the nondrinker, the dietary advice can be followed without relying on red wine as a source of protective procyanidins. A selection of the recipes use polyphenol-rich ingredients to create tasty, nutritious food with that little bit of extra benefit! A two-week menu plan will help you on the way to successful weight control and long-term health improvement.

2

WINE AND HEALTH

IN ANCIENT GREEK mythology, nectar was the drink of the gods. The root of this word means "that which overcomes death." So when the ancient Greeks compared wine to nectar, were they already aware of its health benefits? Around 400 B.C. the Greek physician Hippocrates was using wine as an antiseptic, a diuretic, and a sedative. Galen, a later Greek physician and scholar, further developed the medical use of wine during the second century A.D. He used wine-based medicines and wrote about wine as a medicine in *De Sanitate Tuenda* (also called *Galen's Hygiene*—hygiene in this context means the science concerned with the maintenance of health). In the days before modern manufacturing practices, the use of wine as the base for medical mixtures provided such potions with a degree of stability and cleanliness that could not be achieved with water. Indeed, Louis Pasteur (1822–1895), the French chemist who conducted the groundbreaking work on which modern-day understanding of microbiology is based, said, "Le vin est la plus saine et la plus hygienique des boissons"—wine is the healthiest and most hygienic of drinks.

Over the centuries other notable figures have commented on the health benefits of wine. For instance, in the thirteenth century Arnoldo da Villanova, a Catalan doctor and philosopher, compiled the *Regimen Sanitatis Salernitani* (Salernitan Guide to Health), an early guide to achieving better health. It recommended enjoying wine with meals, but it also taught that wine between meals could have harmful effects. In the sixteenth century Paracelsus, a Swiss physician considered by some as the father of modern therapeutics, is quoted as saying, "Wine is a food, a medicine, and a poison—it's just a question of dose."

australian wine DOCTORS

In nineteenth-century Australia the medical profession was closely linked to the development of some of the first vineyards and the introduction of wine to colonial life. The influence of these so-called Australian wine doctors has lasted to the present day. In 1814, because of the high number of deaths in transit from England, Dr. William Redfern was commissioned by Governor Macquarie to investigate the conditions onboard convict ships. His recommendations to prevent malnutrition and scurvy included a daily serving of a quarter of a pint of wine with lime juice added. Redfern was in fact simply following the best medical practice of the day for preventing scurvy. In 1747 Dr. James Lind, a Scottish naval surgeon, had been the first to discover the importance of citrus fruits for preventing scurvy in sailors. Redfern's wine quota reflected a common belief in its health benefits.

William Redfern started his own vineyard at Campbellfields, southwest of Sydney, and many other doctors subsequently founded wineries in Australia. In terms of their lasting impact on Australian wine production, three of the most influential figures were Drs. Lindeman, Penfold, and Kelly. Dr. Henry John Lindeman and Dr. Christopher Rawson Penfold both trained in London at St. Bartholomew's Hospital (generally referred to as Barts) before emigrating to Australia. I feel a strong sense of their history because of my own links with Barts since 1978.

Lindeman became fascinated by the health benefits of wine on his travels in Europe. In 1840 he emigrated to Australia. Concerned by the heavy drinking of strong spirits in these early colonial days, he embarked on educating his fellow colonists on the beneficial qualities of wine. In 1843 he planted his first vineyard on his Cawarra property in the Hunter Valley, New South Wales. Thirty years later, in a letter to the *New South Wales Medical Gazette* in 1871, he advocated wine as the national beverage for its benefits to both physical health and mental well-being.

Penfold qualified as a doctor in 1838 (four years after Lindeman) and emigrated to South Australia in 1844 with his wife and young daughter. He firmly believed in the medicinal value of wine and brought with him vine cuttings from the south of France, which he planted at Magill on the eastern outskirts of Adelaide. Initially fortified wines were made, mainly for his patients. As demand increased the Magill Estate vineyard and winery developed rapidly. By the 1920s it was claimed that one in every two bottles of wine in Australia carried the Penfolds label.

Dr. Alexander Charles Kelly trained at Edinburgh University before emigrating to the Adelaide area in 1840. He bought land in Morphett Vale, south of Adelaide, and started growing vines around 1845. Kelly became an expert winemaker and wrote an influential book, *The Vine in Australia*, published in 1861, which included detailed information on the best practices in vineyard management and winemaking. In 1862, with the backing of five of Adelaide's leading businessmen, the Tintara Vineyard Company was formed and Kelly was put in charge of establishing the Tintara Vineyard and Winery near McLaren Vale. Despite Kelly's expertise, Tintara was not a commercial success and in 1877 it was purchased by Thomas Hardy. Tintara became the heart of Hardy's wines and remains an important center for wine production today.

While these nineteenth-century Australian wine doctors had faith in the health benefits of wine consumption, and presumably amassed some empirical evidence, we have only recently started to analyze this relationship in detail.

TWENTIETH-CENTURY STUDIES

Medical evidence that moderate alcohol consumption might be beneficial to health was reported in 1926 by the American biologist Raymond Pearl. During his investigations of tuberculosis in Maryland, Pearl found that people who drank moderate amounts of alcohol lived longer than nondrinkers. Pearl was risking controversy with his observations, as they were made during the era of Prohibition (1920–1933). The detrimental effects of excess alcohol consumption were already well known, but this is thought to be the first scientific study showing that moderate consumption of alcohol certainly was not harmful. However, it is possible that other surveys buried in medical archives precede these findings. The cover of a French road map from 1933 (see page 12) suggests others were having similar thoughts.

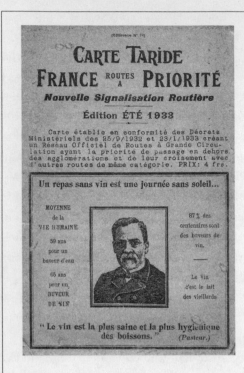

Taride published road maps in France in the 19th and 20th centuries. The cover of this one from 1933 includes testimony to the benefits of wine:

"Moyenne de la vie humaine— 59 ans pour un buveur d'eau, 65 ans pour un buveur de vin' (Average life expectancy is 59 for a water drinker and 65 for a wine drinker.)

"87% des centenaires sont des buveurs de vin" (87% of centenarians are wine drinkers.)

"Le vin c'est le lait des vieillards." (Wine is the milk of the elderly.)

I am grateful to Professor Sandro Capponi of the University of Geneva for drawing this antiquarian map to my attention.

It is clear that attributing health benefits to wine is not a new idea. The question that has caused much debate in recent times is whether all alcoholic drinks confer the same benefit, particularly when many guardians of morality insist that alcohol consumption can only lead to ill health.

THE EFFECTS OF ALCOHOL

When blood cholesterol levels are tested, doctors often advise a change of diet if total cholesterol is high but are more concerned if the level of "good" HDL-cholesterol (see box) is low. A consistent observation with regular consumers of alcohol is that HDL-cholesterol is higher than nondrinkers. This has led some people to conclude that at least half the benefit from alcohol consumption is through increased HDL-cholesterol. Wine, beer, and spirits all have this effect, although the increase in HDL-cholesterol varies from individual to individual, with only very small increases in some people.

Regular drinking of moderate amounts of alcohol also has a beneficial effect on blood clotting. A study published in 1994 looked at the effect on healthy men of drinking alcohol with dinner in the early evening. On separate days participants in this study received 400 milliliters (about 13.5 ounces) of water, 1 liter (nearly 34 ounces) of beer, 400 milliliters (about 13.5 ounces) of red wine, or 144 milliliters (nearly 5 ounces) of spirits; this represented about 40 grams of alcohol for each type of drink. All the alcoholic drinks increased the amount of tissue plasminogen activator (tPA), a substance that activates the clot-busting enzyme plasmin; plasmin acts locally in blood vessels by dissolving blood clots. The increase in tPA caused by alcohol lasted through to the following morning. This was considered an important finding, as it indicates that alcohol consumption in the evening has an anticoagulating action that lasts through to the next day. As a large proportion of heart attacks occur first thing in the morning, this inhibition of blood clot formation may have an important protective effect in moderate drinkers. It suggests that an evening meal that is accompanied by wine is a better choice than just drinking a glass of water.

Alcohol consumption can also affect blood pressure. For a few hours after drinking alcohol blood pressure may fall, but the following day blood pressure is higher than if the person had not had a drink. Because of this "hangover" effect, regular consumption of excess alcohol can become a risk factor for high blood pressure—moderation is key. And drinking alcohol before an exercise test to investigate angina has been shown to worsen angina and increase the severity of electrocardiogram (ECG) changes. So if you have any risk factors for coronary heart disease, then strenuous exercise in a state of inebriation clearly is not a good idea!

THE FRENCH PARADOX

Interest in the health benefits of regular wine consumption has increased considerably over the past twenty-five years. Dr. Selwyn St. Leger and colleagues drew attention to the protective properties of wine when they described an inverse relationship between wine consumption and deaths from coronary heart disease for Europe, North America, and Australasia. Their findings, published in *The Lancet* in 1979, compared figures for men

WHAT IS CHOLESTEROL?

You probably have heard about good and bad cholesterol. Cholesterol is a fatty substance produced by the body; a certain amount is necessary for good health. However, if the body produces too much cholesterol, it can accumulate on blood vessel walls; with time, these fatty deposits may oxidize and harden to form plaques—an early stage of atherosclerosis (see page 20).

Cholesterol is carried in the blood attached to a protein; this combination of fat and protein is called a lipoprotein. Low-density lipoprotein, or LDL-cholesterol, contains a high proportion of fat to protein—this is the "bad" cholesterol, which forms deposits in the blood vessels. HDL-cholesterol (high-density lipoprotein) is mostly protein and not much fat; often known as "good" cholesterol, it is protective through a number of actions. Most importantly, it mops up free LDL-cholesterol in the blood and from other tissue cells and transports it to the liver. The liver breaks down this cholesterol, enabling it to be excreted. HDL-cholesterol is also associated with paraoxonase, an antioxidant enzyme that may protect LDL-cholesterol against oxidation. HDL-cholesterol also has a number of anti-inflammatory effects on blood vessel function. All of these protective effects help explain why a low level of HDL-cholesterol is a risk factor for heart disease.

aged between fifty-five and sixty-four—an age group with high risk of early heart disease—and found the highest death rates were in the traditional beer- and spirit-drinking countries of North America, Australasia, Great Britain, Ireland, Finland, and Norway. France had the lowest number of deaths and the highest wine consumption.

At about the same time, French epidemiologists (scientists studying the incidence of diseases) observed that the French had relatively low rates of coronary heart disease despite high consumption of saturated fat; this concept became known as the French paradox. The idea that regular wine drinking could account for the French paradox shook America when Dr. Serge Renaud put forward this explanation on the CBS television program *60 Minutes* in 1991. The following year Renaud and Dr. Michel de Lorgeril published evidence to support this claim in *The Lancet*. They also put forward the idea that alcohol's ability to inhibit blood-clotting mechanisms underlies this protective effect. Skeptics suggested that the French paradox was simply a statistical anomaly resulting from the way cause of death is recorded on death certificates in France. Hence the question of the health benefits of wine has split experts into camps of believers and nonbelievers.

Media and public awareness of the potential relationship between wine consumption and reduced heart disease was further heightened by a second *60 Minutes* program in 1995. For people who like a tipple, this became the perfect excuse for indulging. But consumers often fail to recognize the fine line between what may have favorable effects and what will cause harm; this is something I'll discuss in more detail in Chapter 8.

DOES WINE OFFER MORE THAN OTHER ALCOHOLIC DRINKS?

Much of the scientific debate over the past ten years has focused on whether all alcoholic drinks confer the same benefit. In 1996, the *British Medical Journal* published a review of twenty-five studies looking at the effect of beer, wine, and spirits on coronary heart disease. Although several studies concluded that wine consumption has the most benefit, the design of many of these studies was considered inadequate for a definitive judgment. The conclusion was that moderate drinking of beer, wine, or spirits lowered the risk of heart disease. The authors of the review (Dr. E. B. Rimm and colleagues) attributed this benefit to the regular consumption of alcohol per se rather than any other component of these drinks. The importance of other factors such as lifestyle and socioeconomic status of the populations were also emphasized.

In 2003, Rimm and his colleagues reported in the *New England Journal of Medicine* their analyses of data collected from 38,077 men in the Health Professionals Follow-up Study. This study includes male dentists, veterinarians, optometrists, osteopathic physicians, and podiatrists aged forty to seventy-five, who were followed for twelve years, from 1986 to 1998. The number of nonfatal heart attacks and deaths from coronary heart disease over this period was recorded. A questionnaire to assess food and alcohol consumption was completed by each participant in 1986, and again in 1990 and 1994. Regular drinkers of alcohol (one to four drinks a day) had a lower number of coronary events than nondrinkers and those who did not drink regularly. Participants in this study were categorized as red wine, white wine, beer, or liquor (spirits) drinkers. Again, Rimm concluded that no specific type of drink conferred extra benefit. What is clear from this study is that having a drink of something alcoholic every day provided some protection from heart disease compared with drinking less often or not at all. This is largely consistent with other studies.

To me it seems of relatively low value to analyze data solely from the point of view of heart disease. The impact of a particular drinking pattern on overall well-being and the likelihood of suffering from any disease is critical for anyone who wants to live a long and healthy life. So the results of two large studies, one in Denmark and the other in France, looking at deaths from coronary heart disease and from all other causes (so-called all-cause mortality) were particularly important. The Danish study was conducted on more than 24,000 men and women living in Copenhagen. Subjects were recruited into the study between 1964 and 1976, and were followed until 1995. The study found that one to three glasses of beer or wine a day reduced coronary heart disease, but only wine drinkers benefited from an overall reduction in deaths from all causes compared to nondrinkers.

Serge Renaud reported similar results from a study in eastern France. Between 1978 and 1983, 36,250 men aged between forty and sixty were recruited for investigation and then followed for twelve to eighteen years. As in the Danish study, both beer and wine drinkers had reduced heart disease. But perhaps the most significant aspect of this study was the finding that wine drinkers who drank two to four glasses a day had 30 percent fewer deaths from all causes compared with nondrinkers or those who drank more than four glasses of wine a day. In other words, the moderate wine drinkers were the healthiest people in both of these populations.

Not surprisingly, excess consumption of any alcoholic drink was associated with a higher number of deaths in both the Danish and French studies—once again emphasizing the fine line between moderate drinking and the risk of harmful effects.

Further proof that wine drinkers generally are healthier came from a survey by Dr. Arthur Klatsky and colleagues in California, published in 2003. This analysis, conducted over a twenty-year period, examined the relationship between the number of deaths and drinking habits for 128,934 people.

Moderate wine drinkers (one or two glasses per day) had a lower number of deaths from any cause; deaths from coronary heart disease were 40 to 60 percent lower. In comparison, regular drinkers (one or more drinks per day) who kept exclusively to either beer or liquor (spirits) showed no benefit in terms of deaths from coronary heart disease or in overall deaths from all causes.

THE IMPORTANCE OF DIET AND LIFESTYLE

Moderate drinking is patently not the only lifestyle pattern that can help you achieve optimum health. The INTERHEART study (published in *The Lancet* in September 2004) examined the relationship between modifiable risk factors and the frequency of heart attack. This study recruited individuals from fifty-two countries and included people from every inhabited continent. A total of 15,152 subjects were enrolled, all of whom had suffered an acute heart attack. For each subject, a corresponding healthy individual of the same age and sex living in the same area was recruited so that various risk factors in the two groups could be compared, to determine which had the greatest influence on the likelihood of suffering a coronary event. A number of interesting points emerged. Not surprisingly, given what we know about risk factors for heart disease, the smoking diabetic with high blood pressure was thirteen times more likely to have a heart attack than someone free of these problems. Regular alcohol consumption (defined as drinking three or more times a week), eating daily fruits or vegetables, and regular exercise each decreased the risk by 10 to 30 percent. Combining all these habits with not smoking reduced the likelihood of a coronary event to one-fifth of someone who did not follow such a way of life. The simple message from INTERHEART is that overall lifestyle is critical for optimum health.

A French study published in 2004 analyzed the relationship between diet and alcohol consumption in the three French MONICA Centers (MONItoring of trends and determinants in CArdiovascular disease) in Lille, Strasbourg, and Toulouse. The survey involved 1,100 men aged forty-five to sixty-four. Diet quality was considered better if consumption of fruits, vegetables, legumes, bread, cereals, fish, lean meat, vegetable oil, milk, and soft cheese were higher than average. Diet was also scored as higher quality if amounts of butter, sugar, potatoes, cheese, eggs, and fatty meats were below average. In this analysis, diet quality was found to be higher for wine drinkers than beer drinkers. Wine drinkers consumed higher levels of fruits and vegetables and lower levels of carbohydrate and saturated fat. Wine drinkers were also less likely to smoke and were more physically active.

Similar findings were revealed by a Danish survey of 48,763 men and women aged fifty to sixty-four. Regular wine drinkers smoked less and were slimmer than nondrinkers and beer or spirit drinkers. Wine drinkers were also more likely to have had higher education. From a dietary perspective, wine drinkers had a higher consumption of fruits, vegetables, salad, and fish, and a preference for using olive oil for cooking. This pattern was most strongly associated with those drinking one to three glasses of wine a day.

By now you may have reached the conclusion that lower levels of heart disease and cancer among wine drinkers are simply due to their healthier and more virtuous existence. With such keen interest in this topic, that would be disappointing! The challenge for me in researching the benefits of wine has been to discover whether aspects of wine drinking really provide something over and above the benefits of a healthier diet.

IS WINE THE BEST MEDICINE?

Serge Renaud has been one of the most influential figures in the world of diet and heart disease. Convinced by results from the Seven Countries Study in the 1960s, which showed the inhabitants of Crete to have a low level of heart disease despite a diet fairly high in fat, he set up the Lyon Diet Heart Study in 1985. This was a clinical trial to test the value of the Cretan-style Mediterranean diet on survival and the recurrence of heart attack in patients who had already suffered one heart attack. Patients placed on the Mediterranean diet were advised to eat more bread, more vegetables, fruit every day, more fish, and less red meat, and all butter and cream was replaced by a margarine provided by the study organizers. The margarine was made from rapeseed (canola) oil. It had a composition similar to olive oil, except that it had notably higher levels of alpha-linolenic acid, the plant source of omega-3 essential fatty acids. After four years, fatal and nonfatal coronary events were reduced by half in those following the Mediterranean-style diet.

As well as looking at diet, the Lyon Diet Heart Study provided an opportunity to examine the impact of wine drinking on heart health. The analysis of wine drinking was restricted to 353 men for whom there was complete information on diet and alcohol consumption during the study. One hundred ninety of these men had followed the Mediterranean-style diet during the four-year investigation. However, when diet was ignored, wine consumption for all 353 men was clearly one of the key factors affecting the likelihood of another heart attack. Drinking between two and four glasses of wine a day reduced by half the number of new heart attacks. This was a very significant observation, particularly as the benefit from wine consumption in this group was clearly independent of diet. It is noteworthy that combined treatment with aspirin and clopidogrel (Plavix), two of the most effective medications for preventing blood clots, only reduces by about one-third the odds of a further coronary event in someone who has already had one heart attack.

For those who enjoy wine every day, the Lyon study gave real encouragement to continue the habit. From the perspective of my research, these data suggested that wine consumption did indeed provide benefits beyond those that could be attributed to a healthier lifestyle and reduced risk factor profile. The observation that even those with heart disease were getting some degree of protection through drinking wine indicated that research to understand these protective effects might provide insights through which new medicines could be developed to benefit all.

STROKE AND OTHER VASCULAR DISEASES

The protective effects of wine in the Lyon study are likely to have resulted from a change in vascular (blood vessel) function. We therefore needed to examine what researchers were finding in studies of other disease areas where abnormal vascular function precedes vascular events such as stroke. We were particularly interested to discover how wine drinkers were affected compared to drinkers of other alcoholic beverages.

People with heart disease are also at risk of stroke. The most common type of stroke is an ischemic stroke, in which the blood supply to the brain is reduced to harmfully low levels. This has many similarities to myocardial infarction, or heart attack. Atherosclerosis (the furring up of blood vessels by the formation of atherosclerotic plaques) occurs not only in the coronary arteries; it may also occur in arteries delivering blood to the brain. When these plaques become unstable and start to break down, they can trigger a blood clot to form that blocks the blood supply to part of the brain. Because alcohol consumption increases blood pressure, it also increases the risk of stroke. So a key question is whether the risks of a glass of wine outweigh the benefits.

Recent analysis of the incidence of ischemic stroke in the Health Professionals Follow-up Study has shown that consuming more than two drinks of beer or spirits (where one drink equals a 12-ounce serving of beer or a 1.5-ounce serving of liquor) on three or more days a week showed a small increased risk. Interestingly, red wine drinkers who consumed one or more drinks per day showed a 40 percent reduction in the number of strokes. This implies that red wine consumption may protect the arteries of the brain from developing blood clots. Since this property was not found with other alcoholic drinks, it suggests something other than alcohol may be responsible for this effect.

Peripheral artery disease is another form of atherosclerosis, which occurs in the blood supply to the legs. It often occurs without any symptoms, but it can be detected by comparing blood pressure in the arm and the ankle. Lower blood pressure in the ankle indicates some degree of obstruction in the leg arteries. The Rotterdam Study of 3,975 subjects aged fifty-five or more showed that moderate alcohol consumption (one or two drinks a day) resulted in a lower level of peripheral artery disease in both men and women. This protective effect was completely lost in smokers. The Framingham Heart Study has examined the relationship between alcohol consumption and the occurrence of intermittent claudication, which is a characteristic symptom of peripheral artery disease. Typically this is recognized by leg discomfort or cramping in the calf during exertion such as walking up a steep incline, which then is relieved with rest. In the Framingham study this symptom was less common in men and women consuming one or two alcoholic drinks each day. Wine and beer drinking were most closely linked to this protective property of alcohol.

BRAIN FUNCTION AND DEMENTIA AMONG WINE DRINKERS

Excess alcohol consumption can have severe adverse effects on mental function. But does moderate alcohol consumption over many years carry any risks for old age? The answer seems to be no; in fact, it's quite the opposite.

There are two main types of dementia: Alzheimer's disease and vascular dementia. Atherosclerotic vascular disease of the brain is the main cause of vascular dementia. So dietary factors that reduce atherosclerosis not only reduce heart disease but also make it less likely that dementia will become a problem in later life.

A study of 3,777 people aged sixty-five or more living at home in the Gironde and Dordogne areas of southwest France has shown that wine drinkers have a lower risk of dementia. Typical of the area, 95 percent of these people reported drinking only wine, the majority of it red. Moderate wine drinking (two to four glasses a day) reduced the risk of Alzheimer's and vascular dementia to about a quarter of the rate of nondrinkers.

The incidence of dementia in subjects aged sixty-five or more has also been investigated in the Copenhagen City Heart Study. Again, this study showed that wine drinkers had a lower risk of dementia compared with nondrinkers or occasional drinkers. Beer drinkers had a higher risk of dementia. It seems unlikely that this was due to alcohol consumption but may indicate other dietary deficiencies in beer drinkers.

In the United States, tests on 12,480 women aged seventy to eighty-one years in the Nurses' Health Study showed that consumption of one alcoholic drink per day resulted in better performance in tests of mental ability. The report on this study in the *New England Journal of Medicine* in 2005 concluded that women with an alcohol intake of a glass a day had a level of cognitive function that was equivalent to being approximately a year and a half younger. A study of male and female civil servants in London (the Whitehall II Study) reached similar conclusions after finding that regular moderate alcohol consumption improved performance in mental tests. In this case the age range of people being tested was younger (forty-six to sixty-eight years). No adverse effects were observed.

Other surveys have also reported that moderate alcohol intake does not have harmful effects on cognitive function. What these studies do not assess in any great detail is whether the lifestyle of drinkers is different from nondrinkers. For instance, it is quite clear from other studies that the more mentally and physically active someone is as they get older, the slower the age-related mental decline. So do alcohol drinkers have more interactive lifestyles that in turn lead to better performance in tests of mental function? Or does alcohol have a specific protective effect on brain function?

The clear association between wine drinking and reduced risk of dementia is very encouraging for all wine drinkers. Whether it reflects a component of the wine or other lifestyle or dietary habits awaits further research.

aGe-ReLaTeD SIGHT LOSS In WIne DRInKeRS

Age-related macular degeneration is the most common form of blindness in old age. Currently there are no treatments available to reverse this condition, a major cause of which is irreversible changes in the structure of blood capillaries in the back of the eye. A number of dietary factors are thought to have an impact on this process, but the effect of alcohol consumption on age-related macular degeneration has not been extensively investigated. Nevertheless, a survey in the United States found that wine drinkers had a lower level of age-related macular degeneration. This may be due to a healthier diet. But, like other observations of better health in wine drinkers, this clearly indicates that the diet and lifestyle of wine drinkers should not be discouraged solely on the grounds that it involves alcohol consumption.

InFLaMMaTIOn anD JOInT DIseases In WIne DRInKeRS

The curmudgeonly gout sufferer is often portrayed as an old man drinking port, and gout (inflammation of the joints, particularly the big toe and ankle) has often been ascribed to excess alcohol consumption, particularly red wine and port. But how much truth is there in this? In the U.S. Health Professionals Follow-up Study, risk of gout was not associated with wine drinking. Regular beer and spirits drinkers were more likely to suffer from this painful condition. Gout was most strongly associated with frequent high consumption of beer, but precisely why this is so is unclear.

Despite extensive searching of medical journals, I cannot find any survey that has compared the level of rheumatoid arthritis (chronic, progressive inflammation and stiffening of the joints) in wine drinkers to nondrinkers. There is evidence that strict adherence to a Mediterranean diet reduces the likelihood of these painful joint problems—a three-month clinical trial of the traditional Cretan diet in patients with rheumatoid arthritis showed reduced inflammation and an improvement in symptoms—but this is thought to be due to reduced meat consumption and increased omega-3 fatty acid intake.

wine, weight, and diabetes

Diabetes and obesity are key risk factors for heart disease, so it is important to know whether alcohol consumption increases the risk of diabetes or obesity. This is particularly relevant when advising people on the best way to lose weight. Most diet plans restrict or exclude alcohol consumption because the calories are considered nutritionally irrelevant and therefore just another aspect of excess calorie intake. But moderate wine drinkers are less likely to be overweight than nondrinkers.

In a French study, the male and female volunteers who drank up to six glasses of wine per day were slimmer than nondrinkers or those who were heavier drinkers. In Spain, strict adherence to a Mediterranean diet, including daily wine drinking, is closely linked to lower body mass index (BMI) and the absence of obesity. A study in the United States found that metabolic syndrome (obesity combined with symptoms of pending diabetes, also known as insulin resistance or syndrome X) was less common in moderate drinkers irrespective of the beverage. The lowest level of metabolic syndrome was observed for wine drinkers.

Several studies have shown that, compared to nondrinkers, regular consumption on at least five days a week of one to three drinks a day of any type of alcoholic beverage reduces the occurrence of type 2 diabetes by 40 to 50 percent. In 2004 a detailed review of such reports noted that heart disease was less common in diabetics who drank a moderate amount of alcohol regularly. The consistency of these observations suggests that it might be counterproductive for someone attempting to lose weight to eliminate moderate alcohol consumption from their diet, as it may increase their risk of diabetes.

Drinking alcohol increases the body's sensitivity to insulin. In some diabetics this may cause hypoglycemia (low blood sugar levels), but often no effect is observed. Reduced sensitivity to insulin is one measure of risk for heart disease; in general, the more insulin sensitive an individual is, the lower the risk of heart disease. A study published in 1998 in the *American Journal of Physiology* showed that in overnight-fasted healthy men, alcohol could inhibit the ability of the liver to synthesize glucose. But the effect was not sufficient to alter blood glucose levels. In diabetics, therefore, whether hypoglycemia occurs probably depends on how recently they have eaten and how well they can compensate for the effect of alcohol on inhibition of liver glucose production. Overall, moderate alcohol consumption with food does not appear to carry any specific risks for diabetics and may even increase insulin sensitivity.

So switching to a Mediterranean diet with a glass of wine with lunch or dinner may improve long-term well-being more than a crash diet that excludes alcohol.

ALCOHOL AND CANCER

It is often said that the increased risk of breast cancer for women under forty drinking a glass of wine each day is greater than the benefit they can derive in terms of reduced heart disease. The Nurses' Health Study has largely removed major worries for the moderate drinker. An analysis of the incidence of breast cancer published in 2000 examined 58,520 women aged between thirty and fifty-five in 1980, who were followed up until 1994. Drinking the equivalent of one glass of wine a day increased the likelihood of breast cancer by 7 percent compared to a nondrinker. This is such a small difference that it seems likely that it may be explained partly by other dietary or lifestyle factors. Based on this study, alcohol consumption was a much less important risk factor for breast cancer than family history, use of hormone replacement therapy, or excessive postmenopausal weight gain.

An overview of the relationship between alcohol consumption and breast cancer, based on forty-two reports covering 41,477 cases, found that one drink a day was associated with a 10 percent increase in breast cancer, which is similar to the Nurses' Health Study. No difference was seen between wine, beer, or spirit drinkers. With two drinks a day the risk increased to 21 percent, which does indicate the need for women to limit alcohol consumption to moderate levels. How alcohol causes this increased risk is uncertain, which makes it difficult to advise preventative measures apart from avoiding excess alcohol. Nevertheless, other dietary habits might contribute. For instance, drinking wine without food leads to higher blood levels of alcohol, and therefore is more likely to be harmful.

In most studies of alcohol consumption men tend to drink more than women. Does this put them at greater risk of cancer? Some reports have suggested alcohol consumption is a risk factor for prostate cancer, whereas others have found no link. Evaluation of information collected through the Health Professionals Follow-up Study indicate that two to four alcoholic drinks a day increases the risk modestly by about 13 percent. But red wine drinkers showed no increased risk. The habit of heavy drinking of any alcohol on one or two days a week was more commonly associated with prostate cancer (64 percent higher risk) than other drinking patterns. Men with type 2 diabetes were also at greater risk of prostate cancer, but this may reflect dietary habits other than just the level of alcohol consumption.

Heavy drinking is linked with a higher risk of mouth, throat, and stomach cancer. This is often associated with other risk factors such as smoking. These uncommon cancers generally are not linked to moderate wine drinking.

Some experimental evidence has linked polyphenols (plant chemicals present in red wine) to anticancer actions, but the significance of these laboratory studies is not yet clear. Diet has such an important impact on the risk of cancer that it is often hard to distinguish between the benefit from wine and the healthy eating pattern of wine drinkers. In fact a diet rich in fruits and vegetables may be sufficient to prevent any increased risk of breast cancer in women who drink one or two glasses of wine a day.

A study published in 2005 in the *American Journal of Gastroenterology* suggested that moderate wine consumption reduces the risk of colon cancer. The findings were striking compared to the increased risk in heavy drinkers of spirits or beer. However, closer examination showed that the wine drinkers were thinner, ate more fruits and vegetables, got more exercise, and were less likely to smoke. These are all habits that are associated with a lower risk of colon cancer, so there may be more to it than just drinking wine.

But for some other cancers wine might have more benefit than a virtuous way of life. According to a Danish investigation of 28,463 men and women, stomach cancer is less common in wine drinkers compared to non-drinkers or other alcohol drinkers. Researchers concluded that a couple of glasses of wine a day might prevent stomach cancer. They also noted that 80 percent of wine drunk in Denmark is red and suggested the polyphenol components of wine might be responsible for this protective effect.

CONCLUSION

Apart from the increased risk of breast cancer in women, moderate wine drinking—by which I mean one to three glasses of wine a day, to accompany food—is generally associated with better than average health. The question for me and other researchers in this field is to discover whether this is primarily due to a better diet or healthier lifestyle, or whether specific components of wine are part of the secret of improved health.

3

WHAT IS IT ABOUT RED WINE?

IN THIS CHAPTER, I'll be looking at exactly how red wine can
help you stay healthy. There's a lot of science, and you can skip
over it if you like, but it explains exactly how my research has
led me to conclude that certain molecules in red wine have a
specific and very beneficial effect within our blood vessels.

Close investigation of the studies summarized in Chapter 2 led many to
conclude that, while regular moderate consumption of any alcoholic drink is
beneficial, red wine is best for long-term well-being. Experimental studies
support this view. In 1981, researchers David Klurfeld and David Kritchevsky
examined the effects of pure alcohol, beer, whiskey, white wine, and red wine
in an experimental model of atherosclerosis (the buildup of fatty deposits in
the arteries). Compared with drinking water, beer provided no protection.
Pure alcohol, whiskey, and white wine had modest protective effects. Only
red wine showed any real protection from atherosclerosis.

Subsequent studies have often made similar observations, but sometimes red wine did not prevent atherosclerosis. This made me wonder
whether all red wines have similar protective potential. If it is a particular
substance in red wine that is protective, then some wines may contain more
than others, and some may contain very little. This could explain why in
some studies red wine did not confer as much benefit as in others. If the
people under investigation in one country were drinking a very protective
red wine, while elsewhere the levels of the protective substance were lower,
then it would not be surprising if the improvements in health were not
always the same. Knowing the active component would make it easier to do

more detailed research into its effects—and eventually might make it possible to produce red wines optimized for these properties or to produce nonalcoholic alternatives.

Experimental studies also indicated that a major component of the antiatherosclerotic effect of red wine was independent of alcohol. Grape seed extract at a dose equivalent to about 1.5 to 2 grams a day was found to reduce by half the level of cholesterol-induced atherosclerosis. Other researchers reported that they had found Concord purple grape juice could prevent the changes in blood vessel walls that trigger atherosclerosis.

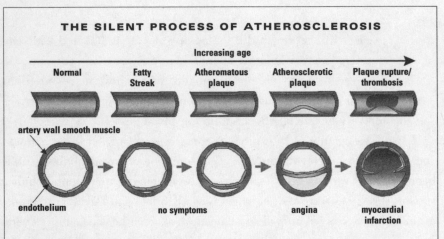

THE SILENT PROCESS OF ATHEROSCLEROSIS

Coronary heart disease develops gradually. The illustration shows schematically a coronary artery, both lengthways (top) and in cross section (bottom). This shows the natural progression of atherosclerosis from early life through to the formation of a coronary artery blood clot or thrombosis, causing a myocardial infarction (heart attack).

Normal healthy arteries can accumulate small fat deposits of bad cholesterol (LDL-cholesterol). This can occur before you are 20 if you eat the wrong diet or have other risk factors. A change of diet and lifestyle can get rid of fatty streaks in the artery wall.

If left untreated, these atherosclerotic plaques progress slowly until they obstruct the normal blood flow and cause angina during physical effort.
Stable angina, although restricting quality of life, is not necessarily life-threatening: some people live with it for many years. The real danger comes from an atherosclerotic plaque that suddenly becomes unstable and ruptures; this triggers the formation of a blood clot (thrombosis), which, by blocking the blood supply to the heart muscle, can cause the heart to stop beating rhythmically, with drastic consequences.

a CLOSER LOOK aT BLOOD vessels

A healthy artery wall is made of smooth muscle cells and fibrous connective tissue. The muscle cells are regulated by nerves running along the outside of the artery wall. These nerves cause the muscle to contract and relax, making the blood vessel either constricted (vasoconstriction) or dilated (vasodilation). Vasodilation relaxes blood vessels, which allows blood flow to increase and blood pressure to fall. Vasoconstriction narrows blood vessels and increases blood pressure. One of the effects of stress—high blood pressure—occurs when the nerves cause blood vessels to constrict. The fibrous connective tissue gives strength to the artery wall so that it can tolerate large changes in blood pressure. This needs to be flexible rather than rigid strength. Too much fibrous tissue makes the artery hard and less able to accommodate changes in blood pressure, so that physical effort may increase blood pressure to dangerous levels. Blood vessels tend to get firmer as we get older, and this increases the likelihood of high blood pressure and other risk factors for heart disease.

All blood vessels are lined with a single layer of cells called the endothelium. This lining creates a nonstick coating between the circulating blood and the underlying layers of smooth muscle. Nobel Prize winner Sir John Vane called the endothelium the "maestro of circulation," because it is a dynamic surface that integrates the interaction between the circulating blood, the wall of the blood vessel, and the cells that make up the tissues of each organ.

The endothelium also acts as a gatekeeper, controlling the body's response to inflammation. As a result of its interactions with circulating blood cells, the endothelium can inform white blood cells where they are needed to fight infection or to respond to other inflammatory stimuli.

HOW YOUR BLOOD vessels keep YOU HeaLTHY

One of the key roles of the endothelium is its contribution to controlling the tone of blood vessels. This is mainly through the release of small amounts of nitric oxide, which causes vasodilation and increases blood flow. In the endothelium, as in other cells of the body, nitric oxide is produced from the amino acid arginine. In large amounts, nitric oxide is a gas. But don't imagine there are bubbles of nitric oxide circulating! The low levels produced by the endothelium remain dissolved in the fluids between cells and in the blood. (Nitric oxide, NO, should not be confused with nitrous oxide, N_2O, an anesthetic, which is sometimes called laughing gas.) Because it has a number of key roles in the body—fighting infection, controlling vascular (blood vessel) function, regulating brain activity—nitric oxide was named "molecule of the year" in 1992 by the magazine *Science*. It also plays an essential role in the male erection. Nitric oxide's vasodilator actions—often referred to as endothelium-dependent vasodilation—are considered one of the most important contributions of the endothelium to maintaining vascular health. Reduced nitric oxide production by the endothelium has been identified as a symptom occurring in people at risk of high blood pressure and heart disease.

The endothelium also produces a number of other substances that are important for healthy vascular function; for many of these substances, the amount produced is critical. Endothelin-1 is a good example. Small amounts are needed to maintain the structural integrity of the blood vessel wall, but in excess endothelin-1 causes vasoconstriction, hardening of the artery wall and—ultimately—atherosclerosis.

Another product of the endothelium is prostacyclin. This is synthesized from a fatty acid called arachidonic acid. Like nitric oxide, prostacyclin is a vasodilator molecule. However, its most important action is to reduce the stickiness of platelets and stop the circulating blood from clotting. Platelets are tiny blood cells lacking a nucleus; they are sometimes described as minute particles circulating in the blood. But platelets are not the lifeless bodies implied by that description. Their main role is to stop bleeding by plugging blood vessels at the sites of wounds and controlling the coagulation of blood. If they become too sticky, platelets can bind to the endothelium, triggering the formation of small blood clots, which may develop into a large clot (thrombosis). Prostacyclin—which reduces the stickiness of platelets—is therefore a key protective factor in preventing blood clots, and if prostacyclin production is blocked, the risk of a thrombosis is increased.

Changes in the endothelium can lead to reduced nitric oxide production and increased endothelin-1, both of which can have serious effects on health. If nitric oxide decreases, then its vasodilator actions are diminished and blood pressure can increase. If endothelin-1 increases at the same time, this triggers even more severe vasoconstriction, which is harmful to the heart. Nitric oxide also has anticoagulant effects on the blood. The loss of normal production of nitric oxide and increased endothelin–1 is called endothelial dysfunction. Research over the past ten to fifteen years has shown it is one of the most common symptoms in patients who later go on to develop heart disease.

Unlike measuring blood pressure, there is no simple way to measure endothelial function. As a result, for many people it goes undiagnosed until they have symptoms of heart disease. Currently there is no medication specifically aimed at treating endothelial dysfunction. So it has become particularly interesting for researchers like me to find that certain substances in red wine seem to be able to restore normal healthy endothelial function.

WHICH SUBSTANCES IN RED WINE HAVE A BENEFICIAL EFFECT?

This is a key question but not one with a straightforward answer. The easy answer is polyphenols—the main contributors to the color and taste of red wine. However, the term *polyphenol* is a scientific smokescreen grouping together a number of substances with very different structures and properties. Phenol is a simple chemical that you may be familiar with from chemistry lessons at school. The term *polyphenol* describes any chemical with more than one phenol group in its structure.

The polyphenols most commonly found in wine are classified as flavonoids (see diagram, page 33); in red wine the most abundant of these are flavanols and anthocyanins. Quercetin and resveratrol have often been used in experimental studies as representative wine polyphenols, but in fact they are minor components of red wine (see The Resveratrol Controversy, page 36).

The flavonoid polyphenols found in greatest quantities in red wine are the flavanols. Flavanols such as catechin and epicatechin are found primarily coating the grape seeds. The higher the proportion of seeds per weight of grapes the more flavanols there are likely to be in a red wine. So grape varieties with small fruit are likely to produce wines that are richer in these polyphenols. Grape seed flavanols are present mainly as procyanidins. When these small polymers (chemical compounds) are composed of three to ten repeated units of smaller molecules, such as catechin or epicatechin, they are sometimes referred to as oligomeric procyanidins (*oligo* is Greek for "small" or "few," *meros* means "part").

Procyanidins are the most abundant polyphenol in young red wines. Initially they may account for 1 to 2 grams per liter of the total quantity of polyphenols, which is usually less than 3 grams per liter. Procyanidin molecules are poorly soluble in grape juice, but as the alcohol concentration increases during fermentation, the procyanidins are extracted into the wine. These molecules are the main source of the mouth-puckering astringency in young red wines. With time these procyanidins react with each other to form longer polymers called condensed tannins. The length of these polymers increases as wine ages. As this happens they become less soluble and eventually form a precipitate at the bottom of the bottle.

RED WINE—A POLYPHENOL COCKTAIL

The colored pigments in wine are anthocyanins. In nature these plant chemicals are the most common source of red coloring in fruits (except tomatoes) and flowers. Some anthocyanins, when bound with certain metal ions, also give blue colors in fruits and flowers. The anthocyanins in red wine mainly come from the skin and are extracted during the fermentation process. Because the juice for making white and rosé wines is separated from the grape seeds and skins before fermentation, there are virtually no seed or skin polyphenols in these wines. This is equally true of white and rosé wines made from red grapes—such as Champagne, which often uses Pinot Noir grapes, and California's White Zinfandel.

Another source of polyphenols in wine is from aging in oak, particularly when new oak barrels are used. Fresh oak naturally contains high levels of nonflavonoid polyphenols called gallotannins; these gradually dissolve into wine after six to eighteen months aging in oak. These substances, plus additional flavors from the oak barrels, contribute to the overall taste and mouthfeel of red wine.

Wine polyphenol composition is very variable, depending, among other things, on grape variety, winemaking style, and soil type. In addition, polyphenols are very unstable molecules. During fermentation and aging of wine, many compounds may be formed through reaction with one another

POLYPHENOLS FOUND IN WINE

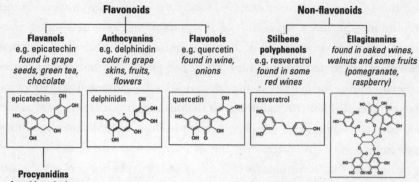

Flavonoids

Flavanols
e.g. epicatechin
*found in grape
seeds, green tea,
chocolate*

Anthocyanins
e.g. delphinidin
*color in grape
skins, fruits,
flowers*

Flavonols
e.g. quercetin
*found in wine,
onions*

Non-flavonoids

**Stilbene
polyphenols**
e.g. resveratrol
*found in some
red wines*

Ellagitannins
*found in oaked wines,
walnuts and some fruits
(pomegranate,
raspberry)*

Procyanidins
*found in red wine,
cranberries, chocolate*

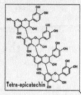

These examples show the molecular structure of just a few
of the thousands of different polyphenols. The most common
polyphenols in wine are classified as flavonoids. The most
abundant flavonoids fall into two main groups: flavanols and
anthocyanins. Of lesser importance are the flavonols (not the
same as flavanols) and the non-flavonoids, such as resveratrol.

O = Oxygen
H = Hydrogen

A PROCYANIDIN MOLECULE

This procyanidin molecule, tetra-epicatechin, consisits of four repeated units of
epicatechin molecules (tetra means four in Greek).

and with other substances in wine such as sugars. Oxidation of polyphenols also occurs readily. These various reactions lead to the formation of a vast number of polyphenolic substances. Estimates suggest that a typical bottle of wine may contain several thousand potential compounds. Many of these are in such low amounts that their precise structures have not yet been identified. These natural modifications to polyphenol structures also explain the evolution of the taste of wine with aging. In the same way that winemakers and wine drinkers rave about both the obvious and subtle flavors of wine that give it its delightful complexity, chemists can become equally effusive over the different chemical structures of polyphenols found in wine.

It is clear that red wines are a well-mixed polyphenol cocktail. So how do they affect well-being, and are some polyphenols more important than others? These clearly are key questions for us to answer if we are to understand whether all red wines have the same potential to prevent heart disease or whether there are wines with specific characteristics that make them more effective.

Researching the Benefits of Red Wine Polyphenols

Research to explain the protective actions of red wine and its polyphenols on heart disease initially focused on two main areas: platelets and oxidation of LDL-cholesterol.

Platelet stickiness is a key contributor to blood clotting mechanisms. This is measured experimentally by assessing the speed with which platelets clump together—a process called platelet aggregation. The action of red wine consumption on platelets has received much attention ever since the provocative article by Renaud and de Lorgeril in *The Lancet* in 1992 titled "Wine, alcohol, platelets, and the French paradox for coronary heart disease." In this report, they described preliminary evidence that farmers from the Var area of southern France had a strikingly lower response in tests of platelet aggregation than farmers in southwest Scotland.

Although research on the effects of red wine and grape polyphenols on platelets has continued, more interest has been focused on their antioxidant actions. Experimentally, red wine polyphenols are more effective antioxidants than vitamins C and E. Could this action prevent heart disease? Many people will know that high blood cholesterol levels are a major risk factor for heart disease. This is because circulating LDL-cholesterol can accumulate in the artery wall under the endothelium, where it becomes oxidized. This is a key trigger for atherosclerosis because oxidized LDL is not readily eliminated. Once present in the artery wall, it stimulates a sustained inflammatory response, which drives the processes of atherosclerosis. If LDL-cholesterol is protected from oxidation, it is less likely to cause atherosclerosis.

Edwin Frankel and colleagues reported in *The Lancet* in 1993 that red wine polyphenols inhibit LDL oxidation. This was completely independent of any action of alcohol and a unique property of red wine and no other alcoholic beverages. A number of studies showed that consumption of 400 milliliters (about 13.5 ounces) of red wine a day by volunteers protected LDL-cholesterol from oxidation. As this effect could not be reproduced with white wine, it seemed clear that the polyphenol components of red wine provided something extra. However, doubts were cast by a Dutch study in which participants consumed 550 milliliters (about 18.5 ounces) of low-alcohol (3.5 percent) red or white wine each evening. The alcohol content had been reduced by evaporation under vacuum. No protective effect on LDL oxidation could be shown. Was this lack of effect due to the choice of red wine (Chianti), or might alcohol assist absorption of polyphenols?

In 1998 the *American Journal of Clinical Nutrition* published the findings of investigations at Papworth Hospital, Cambridge, United Kingdom, in which volunteers consumed 375 milliliters (about 12.5 ounces) of a specified drink every day for two weeks before LDL oxidation was tested. The five drinks were red wine (French Cabernet Sauvignon), white wine with an equivalent amount of added red wine polyphenols, red wine polyphenol powder in capsules, white wine, and a vodka-based control drink. The red wine, white wine with added red wine polyphenols, and red wine polyphenol powder all suppressed LDL oxidation. White wine and vodka had no benefit. So the antioxidant effects were independent of alcohol consumption.

Based on these reports and other similar studies, many people have attributed the antiatherosclerotic benefits of red wine to the antioxidant properties of its polyphenols. But in recent years, clinical trials of antioxidants in coronary heart disease have shown little benefit in terms of reducing the

THE RESVERATROL CONTROVERSY

The focus of my research has been to identify which polyphenols in red wine are responsible for actions on the endothelium. When I started this work several people told me I shouldn't bother because it was well known that the active ingredient in red wine was resveratrol. But some tests in my lab showed this to be unlikely. The amount of resveratrol in wine is typically less than 2 milligrams per liter—a little more than you might get on a pinhead. This makes it a minor polyphenol in red wine.

So why is the presence of resveratrol in wine so frequently cited as the explanation for the French paradox? At the time of writing there had been more than a thousand reports on the actions of resveratrol. It has become accepted as the polyphenol that protects wine drinkers of all nations from heart disease and cancer. This mystified me for years. How did resveratrol become so revered?

*Resveratrol is a phytoalexin. This term derives from Greek—***phyto***, indicating a plant, and ***alexein***, to ward off—and means a substance produced by the plant as a protective mechanism. The amount of resveratrol in the skins of grapes increases because of environmental stresses such as ultraviolet light and fungal attack. Levels tend to be higher in thin-skinned grape varieties such as Pinot Noir; analysis of some (thicker-skinned) Cabernet Sauvignon wines show less than 0.1 milligram per liter. Resveratrol is also found in white and rosé wines, but generally at lower levels than wines from red grape varieties.*

Some of the actions of resveratrol appear to show potential for development as a new medical therapy. Resveratrol can inhibit blood clotting, and has anticancer and anti-inflammatory properties. But there is a major credibility gap between the doses used to cause such effects in experimental work and what might be consumed on a daily basis from drinking wine or eating other plant sources of resveratrol.

In 1993, studies at the University of California, Davis, showed resveratrol could prevent the oxidation of LDL-cholesterol. From this starting point a wealth of knowledge on the experimental actions of resveratrol has accumulated. David Goldberg and colleagues at the University of Toronto have done the most to investigate the actions of resveratrol. In 1995 they described the ability of resveratrol to stop the coagulation of blood. However, the concentration required in blood to cause such an effect was at least 10 to 20 milligrams per liter. Subsequent studies in healthy volunteers failed to show any noticeable effect on blood clotting from amounts that could be achieved through drinking wine. Another study showed that resveratrol could block the early stages of experimental atherosclerosis—but the dose used was equivalent to drinking at least 5 liters of wine a day.

A similar picture emerges from evaluation of studies of resveratrol's anticancer properties. In studies on mice, the lowest dose of resveratrol used was 0.2 milligrams, which is equivalent to a 30-gram (1-ounce) mouse drinking 100 milliliters (nearly 3.5 ounces) of wine—almost a full glass. It is hard to see how drinking, or even swimming in, wine can provide sufficient resveratrol to reach protective levels.

Other research has also contributed to the widespread acceptance of resveratrol consumption from wine as the explanation for the French paradox. In 1997, researchers at the Northwestern University Medical School in Chicago described how resveratrol could mimic some of the actions of estrogen. This was seen as a further argument for resveratrol's key role in the benefits of red wine consumption. Peter Kopp, working in the same division of Northwestern University, wrote an editorial in the European Journal of Endocrinology under the heading "Resveratrol, a phytoestrogen found in red wine. A possible explanation for the conundrum of the 'French paradox'?" This editorial, written to highlight a colleague's research, established resveratrol in folklore. Since then it has been cited in at least sixty other scientific articles as the explanation for the French paradox.

We undertook tests in my own lab to see whether resveratrol modified endothelial function. We concluded that because of the very high concentrations required to see an effect, it would be impossible to achieve these effects through wine consumption. Other researchers have reached similar conclusions.

As long ago as 1997, George Soleas published a detailed review of the known actions of resveratrol in Clinical Biochemistry. From the title of the review one can only assume that Soleas did not hold out much hope for it as the secret behind the French paradox: "Resveratrol: a molecule whose time has come? And gone?" Commenting on the relative inability of resveratrol to cause vasodilation of blood vessels or to act as an antioxidant, he wrote, ". . . resveratrol is a very minor player indeed, and may even more accurately be characterized as a spectator." This represented a very sound conclusion, and there is still no reason to consider resveratrol as anything more than a spectator in the French paradox.

incidence of heart attack. Scientists have gone from thinking antioxidant properties were critical to wondering whether they have any relevance.

HOW DOES RED WINE PROTECT BLOOD VESSELS?

Loss of healthy endothelial function in blood vessels is such a critical event in the development of atherosclerosis that treatments that protect or restore the endothelium to good condition are likely to provide considerable benefit. This also makes it more likely that the actions of red wine polyphenols on the endothelium play a major role in their protective effect.

High blood pressure, raised LDL-cholesterol, diabetes, lack of exercise, age, and smoking all reduce the protective properties of the endothelium. This leads to blood vessels in the heart and other tissues becoming less able to resist the development of atherosclerosis. Whether red wine polyphenols can break the links between all these risk factors and heart disease is not yet known. Experimental studies certainly show that red wine polyphenols protect the endothelium from raised LDL-cholesterol. This supports the idea that red wine consumption provides the explanation for the French paradox—the low level of heart disease in France despite high consumption of saturated fat.

For me the most important breakthrough in our understanding of how red wine polyphenols protect against heart disease originated from studies in 1993 by David Fitzpatrick and colleagues. These showed that red wine and grape extracts caused endothelium-dependent vasodilation through nitric oxide release. Earlier research had studied the antithrombotic effects of flavonoids on the endothelium.

Studies of both healthy subjects and patients with coronary heart disease have provided evidence to support the interaction between grape polyphenols and the endothelium. In healthy volunteers, 500 milliliters (nearly 17 ounces) of red wine—or the same red wine without alcohol (prepared by evaporation under vacuum)—produced endothelium-dependent vasodilation, whereas the vodka drink used for comparison did not do this. It is interesting to note that wine without alcohol was much more active than red wine itself. In another study, patients with coronary heart disease who drank approximately 320 milliliters (nearly 11 ounces) of Concord purple grape juice twice a day for two weeks showed an improvement in endothelium-dependent vasodilation. The susceptibility of LDL to oxidation was also decreased by this treatment.

Studies have also revealed anti-inflammatory effects of wine consumption in healthy volunteers. In one study, compared to no wine or vodka, red wine prevented the adverse effects of a high-fat meal. A second study, a four-week comparison of red wine and gin in men aged between thirty and fifty years in Barcelona, supported the idea of an anti-inflammatory action as well as a specific interaction with the endothelium. After twenty-eight days of red wine consumption, white blood cells showed changes indicating the anti-inflammatory actions of red wine. Blood samples also revealed changes that indicated protective effects on the endothelium.

IDENTIFYING THE VASCULAR PROTECTIVE INGREDIENT OF RED WINE

The history of resveratrol research (see page 36) highlights the problems of extrapolating from experimental research any proof that a single identified factor can account for the beneficial effects of a particular food or drink. Making these connections requires a number of complementary approaches. One obvious point to take into account is that normal intake, for example two glasses of wine a day, provides enough of the identified substance to create the effects ascribed to it. The aim of our research was to discover what was the most important component of red wine for modifying vascular function and preventing atherosclerosis. Through this work we hoped to identify a substance that would provide protection from heart disease.

Our initial experimental studies were driven by various factors. The level of heart disease is very high in the local population of east London, which is the main patient group served by health services linked to my medical school (Barts and the London School of Medicine and Dentistry). For reasons of consumer choice, cost, or religion, red wine consumption is low or nonexistent for most of these people. Even if the benefits of red wine consumption were proved beyond any doubt, wine still would not be on their shopping lists. So the best chance of providing the same benefit might be a well-researched tablet or capsule that would substitute for daily wine consumption.

For people who enjoy wine, there was also the important question whether all red wines provide the same benefit. To me it seems likely that wine-drinking habits could be influenced by knowledge of whether a wine has more or less in the way of protective properties.

Our initial research—published in *Nature* in 2001—examined whether red wine affected endothelin−1 synthesis in endothelial cells grown in laboratory cultures. We focused on endothelin−1 because research over the previous decade had established that this substance plays a key role in heart disease. Endothelin−1 is a potent vasoconstrictor—it narrows blood vessels and therefore raises blood pressure—and triggers processes leading to atherosclerosis. So if red wine suppressed endothelin−1 synthesis, this could then confer considerable benefit in terms of protection from heart disease. To investigate this we tested extracts of different wines to measure their effects on endothelin−1 production. The extent of the effect was closely correlated to the concentration of polyphenols in the wine. All the red wines that we tested suppressed endothelin−1. Red grape juice had less than 10 percent of the activity of the average red wine, but white and rosé wine had no effect. This strongly suggested that the relevant polyphenols were from grape seeds or skin. A number of polyphenols, including resveratrol, had little or no effect on endothelin−1 production, even at concentrations that would have had antioxidant actions. We concluded that the effect was not due to antioxidant properties.

THE PROCYANIDIN BREAKTHROUGH

To address the question of which red wine polyphenols were responsible for this effect, we purified the most potent polyphenols for suppression of endothelin−1 synthesis. Bill Mullen and Alan Crozier at Glasgow University identified the compounds we purified. They were all found to be procyanidins of various sizes and structure.

Interestingly, Fitzpatrick and colleagues had already purified the polyphenols from grape seed extract that caused endothelium-dependent vasodilation. These were all procyanidins with similar size and structure to the ones we identified from red wine. Research into the suppression of platelet aggregation by Concord purple grape juice has also indicated that this is likely to be due to the procyanidin components of the juice.

In more recent work, analysis of a wide variety of wines has shown that the ability of any given wine to modify endothelin-1 synthesis correlates with its procyanidin concentration. Many red wines have a high procyanidin content, with amounts close to 1 gram per liter, which is around a thousand times more than the average level of resveratrol. Only a small proportion would need to be absorbed by the body for beneficial effects to be observed.

AND IT'S NOT JUST RED WINE!

Procyanidins are abundant in several plant sources. This raises the possibility that dietary consumption of these phytochemicals has an evolutionary basis for maintaining healthy blood vessels. The importance of procyanidins and their consumption from different foods, drinks, and other natural sources is discussed in the next chapter.

4

THE MAGIC OF PROCYANIDINS

MANY STUDIES HAVE shown that people who eat more flavonoid-rich fruits have not only a lower incidence of heart disease but also a reduced risk of cancer. Flavonoids are part of the vast family of polyphenols (see page 33), chemical compounds that occur naturally in food. There are many types of flavonoids; they all have antioxidant properties, and this is often given as the explanation for their beneficial actions. However, antioxidant supplements such as vitamin C, vitamin E, and beta-carotene often fail to demonstrate any particular health benefit. Scientists are now beginning to ask whether there are specific interactions between flavonoids and enzyme systems that can better explain the link between a diet rich in natural flavonoids and improved health. Research in my own lab and elsewhere clearly indicates that procyanidins, which are a type of flavonoid, have a specific effect within blood vessels that is distinct from any antioxidant properties.

FOOD AS MEDICINE

Research summarized in the previous chapter has identified procyanidins as the most active polyphenols in red wine. Chapter 7 discusses in more detail how to identify red wines with the highest levels of procyanidins. But drinking red wine with meals is not an option for everyone. This may be for work, medical, religious, or other reasons—and of course wine drinkers sometimes prefer white wine. As we understand more about procyanidins, the question that is increasingly asked is whether there are alternative sources of these protective natural plant chemicals. The answer is, quite simply, yes. Chocolate, apples, cranberries, and certain other fruits, nuts, and spices contain abundant amounts of procyanidins. Starting on page 223, you'll find a selection of recipes highlighting these ingredients.

Procyanidins are virtually absent from grape juice because they come mainly from the seeds and only dissolve in the wine during fermentation. So grape juice is not generally an alternative to red wine. The exception is Concord purple grape juice, which does contain procyanidins (see Box on the following page).

Procyanidins are not the only polyphenols that can affect blood vessel function. Some foods contain polyphenols that we still know very little about. You might find this surprising, but the complexity of their chemical structures has made them hard to purify or study in detail. Pomegranates, for example, are a rich source of many different polyphenols that act within the blood vessels and make a good substitute for wine procyanidins.

Polyphenols of all types tend to be rather astringent, so it is interesting to observe some of the strategies the human race has adopted over the years to develop milder tasting products (the cultivation of less sour fruit varieties, changes in manufacturing techniques, the addition of sugar to fruit juices). Unfortunately, this has resulted in many potentially beneficial foods and drinks having little in the way of protective polyphenols. The best example is chocolate; originally made as a bitter drink, it has become more widely known as a highly processed, sugar-enhanced block of fat with virtually no residual procyanidins. As the significance of procyanidins in food is slowly becoming understood, processes are being adapted to protect these molecules from being destroyed during manufacture and preparation.

If you are a red wine drinker and also eat two or three portions of fruit a day, it is likely you are consuming 1 to 2 grams of protective polyphenols a day. The proportion of procyanidins in this daily quota may vary considerably, but the ideal target to aim for is 300 to 500 milligrams of procyanidins every day. In this chapter I identify a number of foods and drinks with particular benefits for blood vessel health; for each I suggest approximate amounts that would substitute for a 4-ounce glass of red wine. I took as my benchmark procyanidin-rich wine an Argentinean Cabernet Sauvignon that scored ❤❤❤ in my wine ratings (page 105). It has fewer procyanidins than the super ❤❤❤❤❤ wines but is above the average of most modern-style easy-drinking red wines.

As with any sound nutritional advice, variety is important, so even if you drink red wine, eat apples, and add other polyphenol-rich foods to your diet, remember that complete nutrition means eating a wide range of foods. More about this in Chapter 11.

THE LONG HISTORY OF COCOA CONSUMPTION

Cacao trees, which provide us with cocoa and chocolate, are native to parts of Central and South America. The Olmec people are thought to have grown cocoa as a domestic crop on the Gulf Coast of Mexico around 3,500 years ago, and linguists suggest that the word *cocoa* derives from *kakawa*, from the Mixe-Zoquean language spoken at that time. The Maya established the first cocoa plantations in northern regions of South America around 600 A.D. and developed the drink made from ground cocoa beans. Naturally bitter, it could be flavored with vanilla (the seed pod of a tropical orchid), chile, or other spices; honey was occasionally added, but for the most part the Maya did not sweeten their cocoa drinks. From the tenth

CONCORD GRAPE JUICE

Concord purple grape juice has an unusual, aromatic flavor that the wine writer Oz Clarke has likened to "mayblossom and nail varnish"—this flavor is not popular with everybody! Unlike European wine grapes, which are all Vitis vinifera *species, Concord is a* Vitis labrusca *grape. It was developed from native American varieties near the village of Concord in Massachusetts in the 1850s. Dr. Thomas Welch played a major role in the commercial development of Concord grape juice in the 1890s, and it is still most commonly sold under Welch's name. An 8-ounce glass of Concord purple grape juice contains about the same amount of procyanidins as a 4-ounce glass of procyanidin-rich red wine.*

century, cocoa beans were used as currency in many parts of Central and South Americas; this usage continued under the Aztecs, who dominated central Mexico from the fourteenth century until the early sixteenth century. The Aztecs had their own elaborate myths and rituals around chocolate, which they called *cacahuatl*, or *xocolatl*—"bitter water," from *xococ*, "bitter," and *atl*, "water."

In 1502, Columbus was the first European to discover cocoa beans when he encountered a Mayan trading canoe in Guanaja, in modern-day Nicaragua. Although Columbus took samples of these beans, their use and properties were not understood. It was only after Hernando Cortés traveled from Cuba to Mexico in 1519 and was welcomed at the court of the Aztec emperor Montezuma that the use of cocoa beans for making a drink was fully documented. Precisely when chocolate was first drunk in Europe is unclear; some accounts relate that Cortés's gifts to the Spanish emperor in 1528 included cocoa beans and instructions on how to prepare the drink. Others suggest that chocolate drinking was introduced to Europe by a visiting group of Kekchi Maya, who were brought by Dominican friars to the court of Philip II of Spain in 1544. The addition of sugar made the bitter drink more appealing to European palates, and within a century chocolate consumption had spread to most European countries, although only an elite minority could afford it. In late seventeenth-century London, chocolate houses were fashionable meeting places for the privileged few. The most famous of these was White's Chocolate House in St. James's Street, which still exists today as an exclusive men's club.

The cocoa tree was named *Theobroma cacao*—which means "food of the gods"—by the great Swedish naturalist Carolus Linnaeus in the eighteenth century. The naturally bitter taste of cocoa is due to the presence of theobromine, an alkaloid that is structurally similar to caffeine and has comparable properties—it is both a stimulant and a diuretic.

As chocolate consumption filtered down through the ranks of society, changes in manufacturing processes and increasing mechanization meant that chocolate became cheaper and more convenient to make as a drink; chocolate producers in a number of countries also found ways to make "eating chocolate"—a great novelty in the first half of the nineteenth century.

Cocoa beans are one of the richest sources of procyanidins, but modern chocolate manufacturing has evolved to a point where these natural health-promoting chemicals are largely eliminated from the final product. Chocolate manufacture is a multistep process. At each step a large proportion of the procyanidins are lost. After the cocoa pods are harvested and split open, the seeds (cocoa beans) are removed and fermented. This reduces the bitterness, and also the procyanidins—the longer and hotter the fermentation, the greater the loss of procyanidins. The beans are then dried and roasted, primarily to develop the aroma. Both drying and roasting decrease the level of procyanidins. The roasted beans are crushed, winnowed to remove the shells, then milled to produce a sticky mass. Sugar, milk, and other ingredients may be mixed with the cocoa extract to make it less bitter.

Dutching, a process invented by the Dutch chemist Coenraad Johannes van Houten in 1825, uses an alkali to neutralize cocoa acids and produce a milder tasting chocolate. But procyanidins are particularly susceptible to oxidation in an alkaline environment, so this treatment leads to a further loss of these polyphenols.

THE KUNA CONUNDRUM

Since the days of the Maya, some populations in Central America have continued to make a bitter drink from fresh cocoa beans without the sophistication of modern manufacturing processes. The Kuna Indians, who inhabit the San Blas Islands off the northern coast of Panama, are one such population. Professor Norman Hollenberg from Harvard Medical School observed that the islanders rarely developed high blood pressure—unless they moved to the mainland. Hollenberg recognized a link between the Kuna Indians' healthy blood pressure and their consumption of an average of five cocoa drinks a day, prepared on the islands from locally grown beans. This led to involvement with Mars, where Harold Schmitz and colleagues had been working on flavonoids in chocolate since the early 1990s. The eureka moment came when it was realized that the San Blas Islanders' low blood pressure was most likely due to the high procyanidin content of their cocoa drinks. See page 49 for more information on the research at Mars.

The antioxidant effect of flavonoids, such as the flavanols found in chocolate, is well documented, but the specific effect of certain key flavanols—procyanidins—on blood vessel health is a more recent area of study.

In 2003, Professor Norman Hollenberg and his colleague Naomi Fisher published a study showing that flavanol-rich chocolate caused endothelium-dependent vasodilation (beneficial relaxation and widening of blood vessels) in healthy volunteers. In this study, 920 milliliters (about 31 ounces) of cocoa drink was consumed every day for four days; this represented a daily dose of approximately 670 milligrams of procyanidins, and resulted in pronounced effects on vascular function. In a subsequent study, Fisher and Hollenberg reported that the blood vessel response was greater in those over fifty than in younger people. It is generally accepted that the vasodilator effects of the endothelium are reduced with age, and this study suggests that increased consumption of procyanidins could improve vascular function in people over fifty.

Another study described the effect on blood pressure of the consumption of flavanol-rich dark chocolate over fifteen days. Twenty patients with untreated moderately elevated blood pressure were given either dark chocolate or flavanol-free white chocolate. Blood pressure was reduced by the dark chocolate. LDL-cholesterol was also reduced and insulin sensitivity was increased by this treatment. All these actions are encouraging for further research into the benefits of procyanidin-rich dark chocolate.

These reports linking the vascular health benefits from cocoa and chocolate to their procyanidin content reinforce my belief that procyanidins in wine are the key element for protecting the blood vessels of red wine drinkers.

In 2006 the Zutphen Elderly Study in the Netherlands also suggested that chocolate consumption can be beneficial in old age. This fifteen-year study of 470 men found that those consuming an average of 4.2 grams (about .15 ounce) of cocoa a day had 45 to 50 percent fewer deaths than those who did not eat chocolate products. This benefit may be due to flavonoids in chocolate, but other aspects of the diet in this group may have contributed, as they also tended to eat less meat and more nuts.

Chocolate manufacturers are now beginning to make products with increased levels of procyanidins.

In the early 1990s Harold Schmitz and colleagues at Mars recognized that the manufacturing process was responsible for the destruction of many of cocoa's procyanidins. Research at Mars has contributed considerably to our understanding of the actions of procyanidins, and John Hammerstone was responsible for developing the standard methodology by which procyanidins can be accurately measured. After several years of research Mars filed a series of patents for changes in the manufacturing steps in order to retain a greater proportion of procyanidins. The Mars patents are so extensive that they include recipes for various chocolate cookies and other snacks. So beware—if you sell a chocolate brownie you have made using flavanol-rich chocolate from another manufacturer, you could be infringing on a Mars patent!

Products from Mars that use the flavanol-rich chocolate made by the new process are sold under the CocoaVia brand. The initial product was a chocolate drink; in my opinion this had too much added sugar to be considered healthy (3.5 ounces, containing almost 14 grams, or 2 to 3 teaspoons, of sugar). This product is no longer sold, although new chocolate drinks are planned. CocoaVia chocolate bars and snack bars are now the focus of sales efforts, but these also contain a high proportion of sugar (9 grams in a 22 gram chocolate bar).

Mars is not the only manufacturer to have started producing procyanidin-rich chocolate. Barry Callebaut is the world's leading manufacturer of cocoa and chocolate, with operations in more than twenty countries. The company was established in 1996 by the merger of Belgian chocolate makers Callebaut and French-based Cacao Barry. Callebaut made its first chocolate bars in 1911. Cacao Barry originated from an English company founded by Charles Barry in 1842, which first manufactured chocolate in France in 1920. Today Barry Callebaut controls 15 percent of the global cocoa bean harvest and supplies 35 percent of the worldwide gourmet chocolate market. Many major brands as well as artisanal chocolate makers rely on Barry Callebaut for their supply of chocolate. Barry Callebaut has developed the ACTICOA process for preserving cocoa procyanidins. To retain a high level of procyanidins, beans are carefully selected and hand washed instead of using the standard fermentation, drying, and roasting techniques. Chocolate made by this process soon will be available in many countries, but you might not know it unless it is marked with an ACTICOA label.

There seems to be an expectation that procyanidin-rich chocolate and cocoa products are going to take off as a new functional food, with sales worth billions of dollars a year. However, the benefit to the consumer will be minimal unless these are low-sugar products. So if you are going to rely on chocolate to improve your vascular well-being, then you may need to change your taste so that you can give up heavily sweetened chocolate and accept the bitterness of the real thing. Of course, a lot may depend on the outcome of clinical trials in volunteers and patients. If these are successful, then many consumers might find it easier to overcome their dislike of dark chocolate!

Ongoing research of flavanol-rich chocolate is testing the effectiveness of such products for changing the ratio of good (HDL) to bad (LDL) cholesterol, antioxidant status, and blood pressure. Other studies are examining whether these cocoa snacks can improve vascular function in diabetics or in patients with coronary heart disease. Another area of interest is the impact of chocolate on brain blood flow and cognitive performance. In the latter case the combination of improved vascular function combined with the mild stimulatory action of theobromine might prove to be a valuable aid, particularly in old age. In this respect, it is interesting to note that French supercentenarian Jeanne Louise Calment claimed that her longevity was due to olive oil, a regular glass of wine, and eating up to two pounds of chocolate a week. Her wit and lucidity, even at 120 years of age, were widely reported.

a CHOCOLaTe LOVeR'S GUIDe

Some researchers, particularly those based in the chocolate industry, claim that chocolate is universally a richer source of antioxidants and procyanidins than red wine. From our laboratory work I don't believe this can be justified for the amounts that can be found in a normal serving of under 2 ounces. Modern-style red wines are often a poor source of procyanidins, but so too are most brands of chocolate.

Analyses of a range of currently available chocolates and cocoa powders in my lab show that the majority do not contain sufficient procyanidins to warrant consumption for health benefits. Milk chocolate is a nonstarter in this respect. At least 17.5 ounces of most milk chocolates would be required to match the amount of procyanidins in a glass of red wine. Even among dark chocolate there is considerable variation in the level of procyanidins. For some brands you would need at least 4.5 ounces to provide the same amount of procyanidins as a 4-ounce glass of procyanidin-rich red wine; this represents a staggering 600 to 700 calories. Our research has shown that even chocolate containing 70 percent or more cocoa solids is no guarantee of good-quality procyanidins; one manufacturer's 99 percent cocoa solids chocolate had virtually no procyanidins.

In our initial analyses the most procyanidin-rich chocolate came from Ecuador. Among connoisseurs Ecuadorean chocolate has a long-established reputation for fine flavor, but it is also acknowledged as being particularly tannic. People addicted to the sweet flavor of most commercial chocolate will find this astringent taste worth acquiring if they are to gain maximum health benefits from their chocolate habit.

Approximately 1 ounce of a good dark chocolate containing 70 to 85 percent cocoa solids, or about 3 tablespoons of unsweetened cocoa powder, is equivalent to a 4-ounce glass of procyanidin-rich red wine. This amount keeps fat and sugar consumption to an acceptable level and provides around 150 calories. For the very best procyanidin-rich chocolate as little as 0.5 ounces is equivalent to my wine measure. In the future, labeling that includes information on the polyphenol composition will help the consumer recognize the best brands.

The benefits from regularly eating a low-sugar, high-procyanidin dark chocolate in sensible amounts (around 1 ounce a day) are likely to outweigh any harm from saturated fat. In fact, although there is a movement to reduce the fat content of chocolate, more than half of the saturated fat it contains is stearic acid, which is desaturated in the liver and does not lead to increased blood cholesterol levels. The main issue with fat in current chocolate products is the extra dairy fat added to milk chocolate and the hydrogenated fat in low-quality chocolates and chocolate-flavor products—which are all best avoided!

Any health risks from eating a small amount of chocolate are likely to be insignificant in comparison with the importance of regulating total calorie consumption and the amount of saturated fat in an individual's diet.

an apple a Day Keeps The Doctor away

"An apple a day keeps the doctor away" was a common mantra long before everybody was encouraged to eat at least five portions of fruits and vegetables a day. You probably heard this proverb from your grandmother. Its historical origins are uncertain, but it may have originated in Roman times. Did the Romans observe that apple eaters had better health?

Apples contain only modest amounts of vitamin C, potassium, folic acid, and fiber, but recent research has shown apples to be a rich source of procyanidins. Some investigators have suggested that apples are one of the most important sources of these phytochemicals in the U.S. diet. A study

CAN PROCYANIDINS FIGHT CANCER?

Some scientists are now asking whether procyanidins can help prevent cancer. Researchers at Georgetown University, Washington, D.C., led by Robert Dickson, Professor of Oncology, investigated the effect of procyanidins on breast cancer cells. Their study showed that procyanidins purified from cocoa bean extracts, and also synthesized chemically, were able to inhibit the growth of breast cancer tumor cells in culture. This raises the possibility that direct effects of procyanidins on some tumor cells might help reduce the spread of cancers.

Pomegranate juice has also been shown to have anticancer properties in experimental studies. Whether this will translate into a significant benefit in patient studies is hard to judge.

Increasingly scientists are beginning to believe that healthy blood vessels do indeed afford some protection from cancer, possibly by helping reduce the spread of the disease. More research is needed, but it would help explain why people who regularly consume red wine or have diets rich in flavonoids and other polyphenols have lower levels of cancer.

published in 2004 compared the amounts of vitamin C and the various polyphenol compounds found in eight varieties of apples grown in Italy. Typically the apples contained between 10 and 100 times more procyanidins than vitamin C (average: procyanidins, 77 milligrams per 100 grams; vitamin C, 4 milligrams per 100 grams). So a medium apple weighing 5 ounces would provide only about 10 percent of the recommended daily intake of vitamin C but a generous helping of procyanidins. Braeburn and Golden Delicious had some of the lowest levels of procyanidins, although they were highest in vitamin C. For all-round choice an Italian variety called Renetta had the highest levels of procyanidins and good levels of vitamin C. Red Delicious and Granny Smiths are also good choices for procyanidin content but have very low amounts of vitamin C.

It does not follow that if one apple a day is good for you, then two or three would be better. Eating a variety of fruits is more likely to contribute other nutrients. For instance, an apple and a kiwi will provide a good amount of procyanidins (apple) and more than half your daily vitamin C (kiwi). The average procyanidin content of a medium apple is equivalent to a 4-ounce glass of procyanidin-rich red wine. So an apple a day can make a useful contribution to procyanidin intake.

Crab apples have a high procyanidin content. My lab analyses show that, depending on the variety, between 200 and 500 milligrams of procyanidins are present per 3.5 ounces. Crab apples are too small and too astringent to eat like other apples, but when they are in season, adding a few chopped crab apples to a salad could provide a helpful boost to your procyanidin intake.

From my interest in discovering how alcoholic beverages affect vascular function, I have also analyzed the procyanidin levels in a selection of ciders. Traditionally made, unfiltered Somerset cider (a traditional English cider) had a level of procyanidins that was higher than many wines. With only 6 percent alcohol, these ciders make a suitable alternative to red wine. But this is not something that can be said of the more commercial ciders I have analyzed, which typically had between 1 and 5 percent of the procyanidin content of an authentic Somerset cider. Cider, a traditional drink in certain parts of England, France, and Spain, should be a natural product made from cider apples, with little manipulation. Modern commercial products are often made from apple juice concentrates. Fermentation to convert all the sugar into alcohol (7 to 8 percent) means that artificial sweeteners are added to balance the alcohol. And to increase shelf life these "ciders" are filtered to remove all polyphenols, because they can produce a haze on storage, which is thought to be unacceptable. It is no wonder the procyanidin levels are so low in commercial ciders.

As with cider, apple juice is routinely filtered to remove procyanidins. Filtering results in a clear golden brown liquid that can be stored without any further change in appearance. It beats me how such products can be sold as 100 percent apple juice without breaching trade description regulations. Apple juice is brown because some of the polyphenols oxidize during juice making; it is difficult to make apple juice and avoid polyphenol oxidation, so perhaps it is better to just eat an apple a day to keep the doctor away.

CRANBERRIES

Eating cranberries has been associated with health benefits for several centuries. Historically, native Americans used cranberries as a food and a medicine. The preservative properties of cranberries were also valuable in preparing pemmican, an early convenience food. Dried buffalo or deer meat, animal fat, and cranberries were ground together to form a paste, which was dried to a hard, chewy consistency. This provided nourishment on long journeys and during the winter. Early American sailors used cranberries as a source of vitamin C to ward off scurvy.

In recent decades, cranberries have been promoted for their benefit to urinary tract health. They are believed to inhibit bacterial adhesion in the

---

AVOID OVERCOOKING

Because polyphenol molecules are not very stable, when preparing any of the polyphenol-rich foods mentioned in this chapter it is best to avoid anything other than very light cooking—when possible keep cooking to no more than a few minutes. Procyanidins are slightly more stable under acidic conditions, so any recipe using polyphenol-rich ingredients might benefit from a squeeze of fresh lemon juice.

urinary tract, which can prevent or relieve urinary tract infection (UTI) and cystitis. People with diabetes are at higher risk of UTIs.

Cranberries are a rich source of procyanidins, which are thought to account for the protective action in the urinary tract. However, cranberry procyanidins are a different type than those found in wine, chocolate, and apples. So while extracts of cranberry procyanidins have actions very similar to those from red wine on blood vessel function, wine procyanidins do not appear to have the same protective action in the urinary tract.

Cranberries usually appear on the market from October to December; they freeze well, so you can enjoy cranberries all year round. Rinse them in water, then dry them on paper towels before freezing them in 2-ounce amounts. It is not usually necessary to defrost them before use in cooking.

Cranberry juice drinks are readily available in supermarkets. However, it is important to read the labels to make sure you buy a brand with at least 25 percent cranberry juice. There are some 100 percent juices available, but it is not clear whether they have been filtered in a similar manner to apple juice (see page 54). Ocean Spray's cranberry juice is labeled with its proanthocyanidin (an alternative name for procyanidins) content, and it would be helpful if all manufacturers provided this information. The only problem with cranberry juice drinks is the high level of sugar that is often added to disguise the acidity and astringency of the cranberries; I find even the light (reduced-sugar) versions too sweet. During the cranberry season you can make your own juice with fresh berries, using a juicer or blender, and mix it with other fruits such as apples or melons. You can also add fresh or frozen cranberries to mixed fruit smoothies.

Our analyses show that about 2 ounces of fresh or frozen berries or about an 8-ounce serving of juice containing 25 percent cranberry is roughly equivalent to a 4-ounce glass of procyanidin-rich red wine.

Dried cranberries are a convenient alternative to fresh berries and juice. Approximately 2 ounces of dried cranberries is equivalent to an 8-ounce serving of juice, and the added sugar in most dried cranberries is slightly less than the sugar content of regular (full sugar) cranberry juice drink.

However, very few dried cranberry products are the real deal. In 1979, food scientists developed the counter-current extraction technique, which allows the efficient extraction of juice from fruit. It can also be used to reinfuse other liquids back into the fruit residues. In the case of cranberries, the juice may be extracted using this method and the skins refilled with cranberry juice with added sugar or with other juices such as apple juice. It is very hard to identify a dried cranberry that still has all its natural juice and fruit acids.

RASPBERRIES AND OTHER BERRY FRUITS

Analysis in my lab has shown raspberries to be a rich source of various polyphenols. Research by Bill Mullen and colleagues at the University of Glasgow showed that the polyphenols in raspberries contained a high proportion of ellagitannins. Ellagitannins are nonflavonoid polyphenols (see page 33) with beneficial effects similar to those from procyanidins. Using basic analytical methods it is difficult to distinguish between procyanidins and ellagitannins. Our analyses showed that blackberries, strawberries, and red currants contain about the half the level of complex polyphenols found in raspberries; this is still a good level and it is certainly worth including a daily portion of berries in your diet.

The U.S. Department of Agriculture (USDA) has compiled a database of some foods that contain proanthocyanidins (an alternative term for procyanidins). According to this database, red currants, black currants, peaches, pears, plums, and strawberries all have a certain amount of procyanidins. The blueberry's procyanidin profile does not merit great interest and, when cultivated, the fruits are often bland: Their low acidity means the antioxidant

---

THERE'S NOTHING LIKE THE REAL THING

Don't even consider taking cranberry extract in tablets or capsules as an alternative to the real thing. We have analyzed a number of different brands of herbal medicines containing cranberry extract. Compared to most brands of cranberry tablets or capsules, a single fresh cranberry (which weighs about 1 gram) generally contains more protective procyanidins!

components are relatively unstable. This is easily seen if you make juice from blueberries—it rapidly starts to brown because of oxidation. My advice to blueberry lovers is not to stop eating them but to make sure a variety of other fruits are also eaten daily.

Approximately 2 ounces of raspberries—or 3 to 4 ounces of blackberries, strawberries, or red currants—contain amounts of polyphenols similar to a 4-ounce glass of procyanidin-rich red wine.

pomegranates

The pomegranate has a rich history and long association with the medical world. London's Royal College of Physicians features a pomegranate in its coat of arms, granted in 1546.

Pomegranates are native to Iran and eastward to the Himalayas in northern India but have been grown in Mediterranean countries since ancient times. They were introduced into California in the late eighteenth century. There are now many different varieties of pomegranates. Most have relatively soft edible seeds, but some have much harder seeds and may be better juiced.

Pomegranates contain a complex mixture of polyphenols, and experimental studies have shown that pomegranate juice is able to help prevent atherosclerosis. Patient investigations have reported improved blood vessel function and decreased blood pressure with regular consumption of pomegranate juice, so this is clearly a valid approach to improving vascular health.

Our studies show that fresh pomegranate juice has the same potential to modify blood vessel function as an equal quantity of procyanidin-rich red wine.

Two medium pomegranates will yield about 8 ounces of juice. For the best quality juice, use fresh pomegranates and a juicer. Alternatively, use a lemon squeezer: First roll the pomegranate firmly on a hard surface to crush the seeds inside, then cut the pomegranate in half over a bowl to catch the juice, and squeeze out the remaining juice and strain into the bowl. Several commercial products are available, but not all are 100 percent pomegranate juice.

I like to eat pomegranates in a simple fruit salad: To serve two people I use 1 pome-granate, 1 ripe pear, and 1 kiwi. I find the easiest way to recover all the juicy seeds without making too much mess is to cut the pomegranate in quarters, then gently tease away the seeds with your fingers—do this over the bowl so you don't waste any juice. Discard the pithy membrane.

PERSIMMONS, KAKI, AND SHARON FRUIT

Native to China, the kaki, or Oriental persimmon, has been appreciated in Japan and Korea for many centuries. It was introduced to Europe and California in the mid-nineteenth century. There are said to be more than two thousand varieties of persimmon, but essentially there are two types of fruits: astringent and sweet. The mouth-puckering astringency of an unripe persimmon is found in few other fruits. This astringency is caused by a high level of tannins, including procyanidins. As the fruit ripens to a luscious, pulpy goo, the tannins become less apparent.

Persimmons are a good example of how we have developed flavors that are easier on the palate: Sharon fruit, cultivated in Israel, are nonastringent and can be eaten while still firm. In California, both astringent and nonas-tringent varieties are grown. Freezing astringent fruit overnight and thawing the following day is said to soften the fruit and reduce the astringency. It is very hard to predict when kaki are ripe enough to eat but retain a slight astringency so you know there are still some procyanidins remaining. But even when they are overripe and very soft, they are still a good source of vitamin C, beta-carotene and potassium.

NUTS

It was a surprise for the antifat brigade when nut eaters were found to have lower levels of heart disease than people who rarely or never ate nuts.

The Adventist Health Study investigated the link between patterns of food consumption and risk of major diseases in 34,000 Seventh-day Adventists living in California. Those who ate nuts more than five times a week had a 50 percent lower level of heart disease. Skeptics have suggested that the protective effect of nuts is because vegetarians substitute nuts for meat and dairy products, thereby reducing their consumption of saturated fats. But, importantly, the Adventist Health Study showed that the benefit of eating nuts regularly was as great in nonvegetarians as it was in vegetarians.

Nuts are high in fat and protein and are good sources of many vitamins and minerals. They are low in saturated fat, contain between 10 and 60 percent healthy monounsaturated fat and between 5 and 50 percent polyunsaturated fat; in the case of walnuts this includes omega-3 polyunsaturated fat. But there is more to some nuts than a healthy nutritional profile.

Walnuts are one of the richest sources of dietary polyphenols. They are found mainly in the skin coating the nut, which is called the pellicle. These polyphenols protect the fat in the nut from oxidation, although they too will oxidize over time, so it is best to eat the most recent season's nuts, preferably straight from the shells. You will often notice the astringency of fresh walnuts; this is a good sign, as it tells you that the nut is fresh and high in polyphenols. However, if the nuts taste slightly rancid, it means the fats have started to oxidize and the polyphenols are almost certainly past their best.

The polyphenols in walnut pellicles are not procyanidins but a complex mixture of antioxidant polyphenols. In my laboratory we have tested the activity of walnut polyphenols on endothelial cells (the cells lining blood vessels) and found very marked improvements in blood vessel function.

In agreement with our experimental research, a study at the Hospital

Clinic in Barcelona, Spain, showed beneficial effects of walnuts in patients with high cholesterol levels. Participants consumed a Mediterranean diet supplemented with 40 to 65 grams (about 1.5 to 2 ounces) of walnuts every day, either as snacks or in desserts and salads. The result was a 64 percent improvement in endothelium-dependent vasodilation; at the same time LDL-cholesterol was reduced by 6.4 percent. So increasing walnut consumption can go a long way to substituting for red wine consumption.

A serving of 1.5 ounces of walnuts provides an amount of protective polyphenols comparable to a 4-ounce glass of procyanidin-rich red wine. Almonds, hazelnuts, and peanuts contain procyanidins in their skins, and can also make useful contributions to the diet.

Beans and Grains

Pinto beans and sorghum grain, with their brown-pigmented coats, are rich sources of procyanidins. However, finding ways to cook these foods without destroying the procyanidins in the process needs further investigation.

Cinnamon

Cinnamon is one of the richest sources of procyanidins. It is a very versatile spice, suitable for both sweet and savory dishes—it has a particular affinity with apples—so if you like cinnamon, don't hold back! Try sprinkling it on muesli, oatmeal, or plain yogurt for breakfast. See page 229 for my easy-to-make Cranberry and Walnut Bars, which are loaded with cinnamon.

About 1 teaspoon of cinnamon contains the same amount of procyanidins as a 4-ounce glass of procyanidin-rich wine—but that's quite a lot of cinnamon!

Tea

A strong cup of tea is such an astringent drink that many people would expect tea to be a rich source of procyanidins. However, chemical analysis of green and black tea extracts has revealed small procyanidin molecules but not large (oligomeric) procyanidins—the type that can benefit vascular health. My own research has shown that tea extracts have little effect on the function of the endothelial cells lining the blood vessels. Individual flavonoids are abundant, but they have very little protective effect on blood vessel function.

Studies of tea drinkers have given inconsistent findings. In the United Kingdom, where tea is the drink of choice for many, there is no evidence of a reduced level of heart disease in tea drinkers. However, black tea, which has about half the level of polyphenols of green tea, is the most common tea in the United Kingdom. Reduced heart disease in some studies of tea drinkers may reflect their overall better dietary habits than a specific effect of tea consumption. Analysis of a number of studies concluded that drinking three cups of tea a day reduced the risk of heart disease by only 11 percent—rather a small effect compared to the benefits of regular wine drinking. Nevertheless, other research has shown that drinking 900 milliliters (about 30 ounces) of black tea a day for four weeks improved endothelial function in patients with existing coronary heart disease. So drinking large quantities of tea may be a useful addition to other dietary habits aimed at increasing polyphenol consumption.

REMEMBER

This chapter has examined a number of different substitutes for drinking red wine. However, it is important not to focus on a single source of protective polyphenols. The greatest health benefits are gained by eating a combination of foods to ensure that the range of vitamins, minerals, and other micronutrients is as wide as possible. Remember, too, that polyphenols are only a small part of a balanced diet. Variety is the spice of life.

5

DO SIMILAR NATURAL
REMEDIES WORK?

HERE I LOOK at the history of polyphenol research, and also at some of the remedies—extracts of grape seeds, red wine, pine bark, and hawthorn—currently claiming to harness the power of polyphenols to protect against all manner of ills, from high blood pressure to Alzheimer's disease. Do they work? If so, how?

THE DISCOVERY OF VITAMINS

Research into the health-protective properties of food developed from work on vitamins. Diseases such as scurvy (vitamin C deficiency) and beriberi (thiamin/vitamin B_1 deficiency) were for many centuries believed to be the result of infection. In the eighteenth century, the Scottish doctor James Lind discovered that citrus fruits could treat scurvy, but the cause of the disease remained a mystery. It was not until the early twentieth century that scientists recognized the importance of vitamins: A Polish biochemist called Casimir Funk is credited with originating the term *vitamin*, from *vita* (Latin for "life") and *amine* (a type of nitrogen compound). Later work showed that not all these essential micronutrients were amines, but the term *vitamin* stuck.

Much work in the early twentieth century was aimed at identifying the nature of vitamins. The Hungarian scientist Albert Szent-Györgyi won a Nobel Prize for his work on vitamin C, which he had isolated in 1927. Szent-Györgyi was also responsible for discovery of the biological function of the naturally occurring plant chemicals known as flavonoids. Having observed that the capillary fragility occurring in scurvy, which leads to bleeding beneath the skin, was not fully treatable by vitamin C alone, Szent-Györgyi found that flavonoid extracts from Hungarian red pepper or lemon juice successfully restored capillary wall strength. The active principle responsible for this effect on blood vessel walls was given the name vitamin P. In 1936 Szent-Györgyi and colleagues reported experimental studies to support their assertion that scurvy was the result of combined deficiencies in vitamins C and P. The term vitamin P has fallen into disuse, mainly because deficiency states could not be fully demonstrated, which means it does not meet the criteria of a true vitamin. But the concept of flavonoids that can modify the function of both small and large blood vessels lives on. Szent-Györgyi and his colleagues were on to something important. Their research set in train a much wider interest in the search for biologically active flavonoids, or bioflavonoids.

FURTHER WORK ON FLAVONOIDS

In 1947, when Jack Masquelier became a doctoral student at the University of Bordeaux, he probably didn't realize he would become the standard bearer for flavonoid research. He was set to work on discovering whether the red inner skin of peanuts was toxic. He soon showed that peanut skins were free of any harmful effects. In the process he isolated a substance from peanut skin that had strong vitamin P activity within blood vessel walls. At the time, Masquelier did not know this activity was due to procyanidins: A mixture of flavonoids was recognized, but their precise structural identity was unclear.

In the 1950s, peanut skins were not readily available in Bordeaux, so Masquelier sought other sources of this activity. The maritime pine, *Pinus maritima*, grows on the Atlantic coast south of Bordeaux. It is not clear how many products Masquelier tested before he identified the bark of this tree as a good source of the polyphenols he had identified in peanut skins. According to a widely quoted story, Masquelier was driven to investigate pine bark after reading an account of how the French navigator Jacques Cartier and his crew survived the winter in 1534 when they became trapped in

Canada by the frozen Saint Lawrence River. Restricted to rations of salted meat and dried biscuits, the crew developed scurvy. Twenty-five crew members died and the rest certainly would have perished without advice from the native Americans, who recommended drinking a brew made from the bark and needles of a local pine tree. This treatment worked and Cartier and his crew survived.

The scientific record suggests Masquelier's route to the discovery of pine bark procyanidins was less dramatic. In an unembellished report cowritten with Roger David and published in 1952, he cites reports in the 1920s of tannins in other pine species as the stimulus to prepare extracts of various parts of the maritime pine.

In the mid-1950s Masquelier identified vitamin-P-like factors—substances with the ability to act upon blood vessel walls—in wine and cider. This was attributed to the presence of leucoanthocyanins, which I understand by their description to be mainly oligomeric procyanidins (see page 33). In fact, a report in the 1930s had already noted the presence of leucoanthocyanins in grapes. In a review by Masquelier published in 1965 on the role of wine in nutrition, he stated that because of the abundance of polyphenols with vitamin P activity, red wine alone can keep our vascular function safe from any deficiencies. It is perhaps surprising he did not publish more on the properties of wine.

In an article published in the *International Journal of Vitamin and Nutrition Research* in 1979, Masquelier proposed that the flavonoids he had been working on (oligomers of flavanols) should be called pycnogenol. However, this usage did not become widely accepted and the terms oligomeric procyanidins (OPCs) or proanthocyanidins are now used to describe these substances. Pycnogenol is used to describe procyanidins from pine bark, and is a registered trademark for them in many countries. Chemically they are almost identical to those found in red wine or grape seed extract.

From the 1950s through to the 1980s Masquelier deposited several patents on the purification of oligomeric procyanidins and their therapeutic uses. One of these, entitled "Plant extract with a proanthocyanidins content as therapeutic agent having radical scavenger effect and use thereof" (U.S. patent number 4,698,360) became the subject of a classic legal dispute over who had the rights to exploit these inventions. The controversy, with suggestions of fraud and tax evasion, has been disputed in courts in France and the United States, and would merit a feature film if the subject were a little bit juicier.

Despite having assigned the rights to his invention to the U.S.-based company Horphag, Masquelier is involved in the sale of a product called Flavay, a "patented, standardized and genuine oligomeric proanthocyanidins complex" extracted from grape seeds and pine bark. The Flavay Web site claims it is superior to all other products containing procyanidins, such as grape seed extracts. Now, I don't disagree with the view that some grape seed extracts are of very poor quality. I have analyzed several brands of grape seed extract. In comparison with Polyphenolics Mega-Natural Gold grape seed extract (which I use as a reference), most commercial products I have analyzed had less than 30 percent of the expected amounts of procyanidins, and for some products the level was less than 5 percent. Nonetheless, I feel that some of the claims on the Flavay Web site could do with a little more explanation. For example, the Web site claims that this product is based on the scientific methods of Masquelier's patent yet tries to tarnish other manufacturers because they "use chemical solvents which are quite different from water and ethanol." However, the extraction method described in the 4,698,360 patent uses chloroform and ethyl acetate, which are exactly the type of solvents Masquelier implies his product is free from.

THE ACTIONS OF PYCNOGENOL

Pycnogenol is now a registered trademark of Horphag Research. The alleged properties of pycnogenol are so extensive it sounds like a modern-day snake oil. I want it to be clear that I don't consider the claimed benefits of pycnogenol to be flawed, simply inadequately proven. Based on current knowledge of the actions of procyanidins, some of the claims that I find worthy of more extensive testing include:

- Lowering of blood pressure and improved endothelial function in patients with high blood pressure
- Reduced risk of heart disease

- Prevention of blood clots and deep vein thrombosis (DVT, or "economy class syndrome")
- Protection against age-related eye diseases and sight loss

Other alleged properties where I am less convinced but wouldn't exclude some benefit are:

- Prevention of Alzheimer's disease; improvement of memory
- Reduced risk of cancer
- Anti-inflammatory
- Reduced arthritis symptoms
- Beneficial effects on asthma and chronic bronchitis
- Inhibition of menstrual cramps; reduced symptoms of endometriosis
- Improvement of skin conditions; psoriasis treatment; wrinkle prevention

One condition that is missing from this list that I think could be included is erectile dysfunction. Vascular malfunction is a major factor in this problem and, based on the known actions of procyanidins, it is plausible that erectile dysfunction would respond to treatment with pycnogenol. This omission is surprising because claims of efficacy in this area usually boost a product's sales. But getting the daily dose right will require careful optimization before pycnogenol can be claimed to be the natural Viagra.

There have been a number of small-scale clinical trials using pycnogenol. Many of the findings are positive and in agreement with what is known about the actions of procyanidins through experimentation. But then why has pycnogenol not entered mainstream medical practice? It seems that Horphag Research has been unwilling to test it in a large-scale double-blind outcome study to show that it really works. These clinical trials are routinely undertaken by pharmaceutical companies. Neither the patient nor the doctor knows who is receiving the active medication or an inactive placebo. Such a trial runs for a fixed period of a few months to a few years, depending on the disease and the medication being studied. At the end of the study the patients who showed an improvement in their condition or symptoms are counted to see if there is a significant benefit compared to the inactive placebo. Studies may involve several thousand people to observe whether there is any significant benefit over what may happen by chance, because some patients may see an improvement in their symptoms over time even without treatment. A range of doses also needs to be tested to find the best dose for conferring benefit without causing side effects.

Purveyors of herbal medicines and other complementary therapies are often reluctant to do this type of clinical trial. This is basically for two reasons: cost and risk. The cost of such trials is usually prohibitive for small companies. The risk is that the treatment doesn't prove to be effective in the trial. In that case the company would no longer be able to promote it as suitable for the range of illnesses they would like to think it might benefit. However, if successful the product could become a prescription medication, which would make a big difference to its commercial value. So with the evidence that Horphag has accumulated, it is surprising that it has not taken the decision to undertake at least one large-scale clinical trial.

The beneficial effects of pycnogenol have been attributed to the antioxidant activity of procyanidins. This is based on Masquelier's 4,698,360 patent, which claimed protective actions in Alzheimer's disease, atherosclerosis, cancer, and any inflammatory disease linked to free radical damage. If all the claims were true, describing pycnogenol as a panacea for contemporary ills would not be out of place. However, I don't think there has yet been a sufficiently rigorous assessment of pycnogenol's ability to alleviate symptoms or an adequate evaluation of the ideal dose for each of the claimed actions. In my opinion, the full potential for pycnogenol will not be realized while its effects are linked to some nebulous superantioxidant property.

In the past ten years, procyanidins have been shown to have a number of effects on blood vessel function that are unrelated to antioxidant activity. Furthermore, procyanidins from different sources have been shown to have a positive interaction with platelets (tiny blood cells that, if they become too sticky, can trigger the formation of blood clots and may lead to thrombosis); this is an important protective effect in heart disease. In fact, a U.S. patent (5,720,956) has been awarded for this action of pycnogenol. This might be one of the most important uses for procyanidins (whatever their origin), and could be the best opportunity for a large-scale clinical trial to fully test the power of pycnogenol.

In terms of likely benefit to the consumer, capsules of red wine extract are the most ludicrous product I have analyzed. There are several different wine extracts sold in the United States and Europe that are promoted as alcohol-free alternatives to wine. I'm not convinced they are good value. For one product I tested each capsule contained the equivalent of about half a teaspoon of procyanidin-rich wine. For the price of thirty capsules you could buy a very nice bottle of red wine, and even if you were to drink a teaspoon a day, it would be better value than the capsules.

HAWTHORN EXTRACT—A TRADITIONAL REMEDY FOR HEART FAILURE

Hawthorn extract is a popular herbal remedy in the United States and Europe. In Germany it is available as a prescription medication. It is prepared from *Crataegus monogyna* or *Crataegus laevigata*, either as extracts of leaves and flowers, or from berries. As far as I know, this is the only medicine found in the European Pharmacopoeia whose characteristics are defined by the level of procyanidins. Experimental studies have shown it improves blood flow through the coronary arteries, and therefore increases the amount of blood reaching the heart muscle. This is in agreement with observations that it increases the efficiency of contraction of the heart. Clinical studies in patients with heart failure have shown improved cardiac function, increased exercise tolerance, and a decrease in heart failure–related symptoms, without any apparent side effects.

The historical use of hawthorn extract as an herbal medicine for heart failure highlights the potential that dietary sources of procyanidins might have for preventing symptoms of this condition. Heart failure occurs progressively to some extent in everybody in old age. Typical symptoms might be a cough or breathlessness at night due to accumulation of fluid in the lungs when lying down, and swelling of the ankles during the day. Difficulty in walking any distance, particularly uphill, without becoming breathless may also be an indication of some degree of heart failure. If you regularly suffer from these symptoms, you should get checked over by your doctor.

Why does heart failure occur as we get older? The heart muscle may become stiffer and pump less efficiently. The blood supply to the heart muscle may be reduced because of atherosclerotic lesions partially blocking the coronary arteries. Blood vessels become less flexible with age, and this increases the resistance the heart has to pump against, which increases the effort required for the heart to pump blood around the body. It appears that procyanidins from hawthorn extract and other sources help by improving blood flow to the heart and by causing vasodilation of other blood vessels. This helps the heart pump more effectively and decreases its workload. The result is a decrease in symptoms.

The degree of benefit from hawthorn extract in heart failure might depend on the severity of the disease at the start of treatment. A study by Professor Michael Tauchert in Germany showed hawthorn extract had beneficial effects on patients with advanced chronic heart failure. The extract used was standardized to contain 18.75 percent procyanidins. After sixteen weeks of treatment, improvement in symptoms and an increase in maximum tolerated workload during exercise were observed in patients taking 1800 milligrams of this extract a day, which represents approximately 340 milligrams of procyanidins. No benefit was observed in patients taking half this dose. So to see improvements in patients with heart failure, the dose is of critical importance.

PROTECTIVE PROCYANIDINS

Tauchert's study was on patients with fairly severe heart failure. If large amounts of procyanidins were consumed daily over many years, would this reduce the likelihood of heart failure occurring in the first place? I found this interesting because of my research on the Italian island of Sardinia, where there were an unusual number of centenarians living in Nuoro province. Might their longevity be due to other dietary sources of procyanidins? Sardinians in Nuoro who drink about half a bottle (375 milliliters) a day of the tannic local wine would have an intake of procyanidins (250 to 350 milligrams) similar to the dose of hawthorn extract administered in Tauchert's study. So perhaps the procyanidin-rich wines have been instrumental in helping these people live longer by providing protection from both atherosclerosis and heart failure, two major causes of death in the modern world.

The large dose of hawthorn extract that was required before any benefit was observed in patients with heart failure emphasizes the need for more research on the optimal daily dose of supplements containing procyanidins. It seems to me that commonly used doses of 50 to 100 milligrams of procyanidins—whether as hawthorn extract, pycnogenol, or grape seed extract—are unlikely to confer the maximal achievable benefit. Further research and clinical trials are needed to allow a better definition of the optimal daily amount of procyanidins to consume for beneficial changes in heart function.

6

eaT, DRINK, and Be HeaLTHY aT 100 YeaRS OLD

WILL YOU LIVE to be 100? Will you be healthy enough to enjoy your hundredth birthday? In some societies this is considered both reasonable and achievable. In Sardinia, for instance, the common greeting "A kent'annos"—"to one hundred years"—is often answered with "may you live to count the years." Apparently this wish often comes true: Sardinia's mountainous Nuoro province is reported to have the highest relative number of centenarians in Europe, even though these remote parts of the island have nothing more than rudimentary medical care. So what is it about their diet and lifestyle that underlies the exceptional aging of the Nuoresi?

What can we learn about people who have longer-than-average life expectancies? Is it their genes? Where they live? The food they eat, or what they drink? Are there other aspects of their daily habits and lifestyle that protect them from common age-related diseases? Can we obtain insights for improving our diet and lifestyle by looking at populations where the level of heart disease and cancer is lower or occurs later in life? The answer to this last question is almost certainly yes.

Current lifestyle habits are without doubt shortening lives in many countries. The average life expectancy in the United States is thought to be ten years less than it should be because too many people smoke, 75 percent are overweight or obese, and few people take daily exercise. Yet how many centenarians in Nuoro have access to a fitness center now, let alone fifty years ago? Short bursts of intense exercise in the gym may not be the ideal substitute for the traditional activities and other daily habits of these Sardinians.

UNDERSTANDING LONGEVITY

Scientists studying the processes of aging frequently claim that medical advances will soon raise life expectancy to at least 100 years. However, given the high cost of treatments such as stem cell implants for a failing heart or for restoration of brain function, it is unlikely that many people will benefit. To help more people live longer and remain healthy and active in old age will require further research on the prevention of common age-related diseases. This would be a wider-reaching, more cost-effective approach than expecting to provide everybody with complex new therapies. Only then will the number of elderly people increase without overburdening health care resources.

Current research is focused on three main questions:

- What is the maximum possible life span for humans?
- How much do genes contribute to longevity?
- What are the lifestyle factors that have the most influence on long-term survival?

The last of these is the most important, because it is the only aspect that we can modify to change our life expectancies.

Recent estimates suggest that there are about 200,000 centenarians worldwide, and this number is expected to grow to three million by 2050 provided there is not a pandemic of deadly influenza or other highly infectious illness. Some researchers have now turned their attention to super-centenarians—people aged 110 or more. No more than 300 to 400 people worldwide fall into this group; in fact, during the past ten years at any given time there have been fewer than fifty fully validated supercentenarians. Investigations of people claiming to have reached the age of 110 have often found a lack of accurate records to support the claim or have shown the declaration to be false.

The longest-lived person ever—verified by *The Guinness Book of Records*—was a French woman, Jeanne Louise Calment, who died on August 4, 1997, aged 122 years and 164 days. Some might imagine that it is only a matter of time before this record is exceeded, but very few centenarians live past 115 years of age, and it is unlikely that this record will be broken at any time in the near future without considerable assistance from medical science. Perhaps sponsors of research into aging will offer prizes for insights enabling people to live to this age. But the greater the incentive the more likely there will be fakes.

THE GENETICS OF LONGEVITY

For many people there is no relationship between their age at death and that of their parents. But in families with many members regularly living into their nineties or more there is a much closer relationship between the life span of parents and their children. It is highly likely that genes are playing a part in such cases. Most experts think that the genetics of longevity is a complex interaction between genes that favor a slower rate of aging and genes that influence susceptibility to age-related illnesses—or the absence of genes that put individuals at risk of disease. The importance of genetic factors in relation to certain illnesses is clear. Surveys have shown that the offspring of centenarians have approximately half the level of diabetes and heart disease when compared with other people of the same age.

Approximately 85 percent of centenarians are women. While some centenarians reach such an age only through medical intervention, others may have had no major illness. To address the question of how genes contribute to longevity, J. Evert and colleagues examined the medical histories of centenarians and used these as a basis for their classification into "Survivors," "Delayers," and "Escapers":

- Survivors are those who had diseases such as heart disease or cancer before they were eighty but thanks to medical interventions managed to live to 100.
- Delayers have also suffered from age-related diseases such as heart disease and cancer, but the onset of disease was delayed until they were eighty or older.
- Escapers have lived to this age free of common age-related disorders.

CATEGORIES OF CENTENARIANS

	MALE (PERCENT)	FEMALE (PERCENT)
Survivors	24	43
Delayers	44	42
Escapers	32	15

(Adapted from Evert and colleagues, 2003)

The most interesting group in terms of studying the genetic factors and lifestyle influences enabling a person to live to 100 years of age are the Escapers. But extensive probing into Escapers' lives and habits does not reveal anything unusual that could be considered to have protected them from disease. Of course, it is hard to identify the different aspects of a lifestyle that have had the greatest influence over 100 years of life. A snapshot of habits in someone's latter years may miss key factors in early life. So often we are left thinking that genetics play a major part.

Despite these difficulties in defining what influences longevity, some scientists still claim that unlimited life expectancy is only a matter of time. With our current knowledge of aging processes I think it is extremely doubtful that this will be achieved in the lifetime of these scientists. Life expectancy is increasing in many countries, but there is no real evidence that maximum life span is showing similar increases. Indeed, the idea that there will be a time with no limits to human life span completely misrepresents current facts and scientific understanding.

Although it is considered unlikely that a single gene that increases longevity will be found, this has not stopped scientists from hunting for such genes. Those who hope to find the genetic answer to extending life indefinitely have to date studied yeasts, fruit flies, and nematode worms. It is fairly easy to do these experiments and live to see the results because the maximum life spans for these species are weeks or months rather than years. The common approach used to study the role played by specific genes is to selectively inactivate a gene and see what happens. The alternative approach is to make a gene overactive to see how that affects life span. These experiments are a long way from extrapolation to the human scale. Even if key genes that influence longevity can be identified, ways of turning these genes on or off in humans will also need to be discovered. So creation of a modern-day Methuselah is still a long way off (according to the Bible, Methuselah lived 969 years—Genesis 5: 21–27).

VOODOO SCIENCE IN THE STRUGGLE TO STAY YOUNG

Many people are more concerned with hiding the signs of aging than making lifestyle changes that might ensure a longer life. Antiaging therapies offer their promoters the opportunity to make large amounts of money; youth-prolonging claims are already being made for high-dose vitamin therapies. Some of these products may indeed have some benefit. But the claims for these remedies are not based on long-term clinical trials, or on population studies linking the proposed therapy with long-lived individuals. Far more could be achieved through other, longer-term, lifestyle changes.

The whole subject of aging has become crowded by voodoo science. This term refers to science that is not proven to any point of certainty. However, if it is repeated often enough—the voodoo chant—then everybody starts to believe it to be true. Voodoo science doesn't just confuse the nonscientist; even scientists sometimes seem to lose their ability to critically appraise their work. The most repeated voodoo chant in this area is that aging can be prevented by increased consumption of antioxidants.

YOUR ANTIOXIDANT DEFENSE SYSTEM

Most research points to oxidative stress as a trigger for accelerating the aging processes. Oxidative stress occurs when highly reactive forms of oxygen, sometimes referred to as free radicals, damage proteins and DNA. With prolonged oxidative stress, damage to cells accumulates and cells either fail to function properly or die. So the current voodoo chant is that aging processes can be easily prevented by consumption of large quantities of antioxidants, such as beta-carotene, vitamin C, and vitamin E. But large-scale clinical trials of high-dose antioxidant therapies have generally shown no benefit. In some cases, supplements may even be harmful, as people following these nostrums have survived less well than those receiving no treatment.

You might be wondering how that is possible. Well, the body relies on a natural balance between pro-oxidant and antioxidant mechanisms. The body's ability to fight infection and kill cancer cells is dependent on reactive oxygen, or free radicals. Healthy cells have their own antioxidant defense mechanisms, which become active when cells are exposed to pro-oxidant stresses. High doses of antioxidants can prevent these defense mechanisms from working properly, which may lead to less protection for some cells than if these "protective" vitamins were not taken. So the most important goal for everyone is to achieve the right balance of vitamins, minerals, and other micronutrients. A vitamin supplement may be helpful for some people if their diet is inadequate, but very high dose supplements are unlikely to provide a magic cure to the processes of aging.

The theory that increasing antioxidant defenses is a good idea is not wrong. The issue is how this is achieved. Each cell in the body contains tiny structures called mitochondria, which are responsible for turning glucose and other fuels into energy—imagine tiny furnaces burning rapidly with sparks flying. When the energy-making processes are in full swing, then reactive oxygen (free radicals) that causes oxidative stress can be inadvertently produced. Mitochondria normally stop these free radicals from causing damage through defense mechanisms that rapidly inactivate them. What appears to happen with aging is that these defense mechanisms are not sufficiently protective. Genetic modifications of mice and fruit flies have shown it is possible to increase their life spans through changing the function of specific genes that increase protection from oxidative stress. These protective genes work by making proteins that mop up free radicals before they do any damage. Why these proteins are effective when antioxidants are not could be because their activity is restricted to parts of cells where increased protection is required.

A study published in 2005 in the journal *Science* showed that a selective increase in activity of a protective enzyme called catalase increased the life span of mice by about 20 percent. Not only was life span increased, but also signs of aging in the heart, such as arteriosclerosis, were decreased. This worked only when the catalase activity was increased in the mitochondria and not in other parts of the cell. So to slow aging processes, rather than consuming large quantities of antioxidant vitamins, we need to find ways of increasing the level of protection from our natural antioxidant defense system.

CALORIE RESTRICTION AS A STRATEGY
TO INCREASE LIFE SPAN

In laboratory studies researchers have consistently observed that calorie restriction can increase life span. There is considerable interest in what long-term benefits can be demonstrated in human subjects willing to follow this type of extreme diet. This led to the formation in the mid-1990s of a Calorie Restriction Society in the United States whose aim is to extend life span by reducing calorie intake while maintaining adequate nutrition. In laboratory animals, calorie restriction is generally not effective when initiated in later life. The only exception appears to be for cancer-prone strains of mice where a decreased occurrence of tumors on calorie restriction increases the average life span. For humans the point at which calorie restriction might be most beneficial has yet to be defined. Certainly such a strategy would be expected to reduce the likelihood of diabetes and slow the progression of heart disease, so some benefit is likely. Luigi Fontana and colleagues confirmed this in 2004 when they reported that blood pressure and other risk factors for heart disease were much lower in subjects pursuing a regime of long-term calorie restriction.

If you want further encouragement to go down this route, then you will be pleased to know that there are studies showing leaner people have the longest life expectancies, which indirectly supports the benefits of calorie restriction. Two reports, one on men and another on women, showed that individuals with a body weight 15 to 20 percent below average had the lowest mortality, provided their lower weight was not due to illness or smoking.

People living in the Okinawa islands of Japan are said to have the longest average life span in the world. This is attributed in part to their diet, which is lower in calories than the average diet in Japan—and substantially lower than that in most parts of North America and Europe. A typical Okinawan diet is composed mainly of abundant vegetables, protein from vegetable sources or fish, and carbohydrate from rice or potatoes. Physical activity may also be an important factor. Agriculture was the main occupation of Okinawan centenarians, who had often worked into their seventies.

Calorie restriction is not without its problems, which include low blood pressure (which may causing fainting), loss of libido and infertility, osteoporosis, loss of muscle strength, and, not surprisingly, low energy levels! If that isn't bad enough, irritability and depression can affect those pursuing calorie restriction, which all sounds rather hard to live with if you want a full and active life.

Research to identify the protective mechanisms activated by calorie restriction is under way. If these mechanisms can be activated by other means, then it is possible that some of the effects of calorie restriction could be mimicked without greatly reducing food intake. I am not aware of any studies showing that calorie restriction increases antioxidant defenses, so the effects of calorie restriction may be unrelated to oxidative stress as an explanation for aging. However, decreased metabolic activity due to calorie restriction may simply decrease free radical production by mitochondria so that the burden on antioxidant defense mechanisms is less.

I do not recommend extreme calorie restriction as a strategy to increase longevity; there is a real danger of malnutrition if the diet is not carefully balanced. A simple reduction in the intake of calorie-rich foods to reach optimal body weight is potentially just as effective and certainly more achievable in the longer term.

SEEKING THE FOUNTAIN OF ETERNAL YOUTH

How can we learn which diet and lifestyle is best to ensure maximum longevity for the set of genes we inherited from our parents? To get a balanced picture, the only feasible approach is to study people who live in good health into old age, even if they don't all become centenarians. Too much focus on the types of food and other habits of a few centenarians who have gone through life without major disease (the Escapers—see page 76) may make it difficult to separate the lifestyle from the genes. This is particularly true when exercise-avoiding, slightly overweight former smokers are put forward as examples of people who have lived to become centenarians despite their lifestyle.

My interest in factors affecting longevity developed from observations that moderate wine drinkers had an overall lower number of deaths over the period of the studies. Was this due to the wine or the generally healthier lifestyles of wine drinkers? If the wine drinkers had a lower number of deaths, do they live longer on average? This is a difficult question to answer because this type of investigation rarely follows each person until they eventually breathe their last. How could I solve this conundrum? I came up with an alternative approach—to investigate whether wine drinkers who lived the longest were drinking wine with particular properties. Sardinia seemed a good place to start such investigations, as I was aware that an unusual number of centenarians lived on the island. Also, at the time of my initial interest in Sardinian centenarians, the oldest man in the world was Antonio Todde, who lived in the Sardinian town of Tiana. He died a few weeks short of his 113th birthday in January 2002.

I sought backing from several sources to investigate the relationship between the local wines and longevity in Sardinia. The Geoffrey Roberts Award committee selected my project for funding, and this led to my trip in the summer of 2002 to study whether the wines of Sardinia had special properties.

SARDINIAN CENTENARIANS

Sardinia is not entirely typical of Mediterranean islands. It is a large island—only Sicily is bigger. Over the generations, what probably has been most important for the lifestyle and gene pool of the people of Sardinia is its remoteness. Although there have been invaders over the centuries, they rarely entered the mountainous eastern areas.

Professor Luca Deiana at the University of Sassari leads the AKEA study of extreme longevity in Sardinia. The name AKEA comes from the traditional Sardinian salutation of "A kent'annos" mentioned at the start of this chapter. Initially, Deiana's research team mapped the centenarians living in Sardinia and verified their dates of birth. This revealed a higher number of centenarians than in other European countries (more than 16 per 100,000 people, compared to an average of 10 per 100,000). Surprisingly, the female to male ratio was only 2 to 1, as this ratio is typically more than 5 to 1. Further investigation showed extreme longevity in Sardinia was concentrated in the mountainous central-eastern part of the island. This became known as the Blue Zone in reference to the blue marker pen used to map the location of centenarians. These mountains have been known for centuries as the Gennargentu ("silver gate," from the Latin *Janua argenti*). In ancient times this area was a refuge for the Sardinian locals from invaders such as the Romans, who called it Barbaria because it was never brought under their control. This is the origin of Barbagia, the current name for much of this area.

The Blue Zone covers the mountainous region of Sardinia's Nuoro province. In 2002 the central area of the Blue Zone had forty-seven male centenarians and forty-four female centenarians (a female to male ratio of 0.94 to 1). This is quite remarkable, and it implies unusual benefit to men from the underlying environmental, lifestyle, or genetic factors. Access to this area's remote towns and villages is via some very steep and twisty roads, and for generations the communities here were virtually cut off from outside influences. This is considered a good argument for genetic factors underlying this unusual longevity. The remoteness limited the number of people moving into the area, so intermarrying between related families is likely to have led to a restricted gene pool. The consequence of this could be that any genes that favored longevity or protection from common diseases such as heart disease would have become common in this population.

When I visited Professor Deiana and his colleague Dr. Giovanni Pes in the summer of 2002, they were highly skeptical that wine had any influence on longevity in these centenarians. But they also admitted that they had not been able to identify a genetic link. So an environmental or lifestyle factor could be important. Interestingly, the typical diet in Professor Deiana's Blue Zone is not what I had anticipated. Unlike the typical Mediterranean eating pattern, it was fairly low in vegetables, and fish was not a central part of the diet. I was told that in the past the coast was so difficult to reach that it was almost impossible to bring fish into the mountains and keep it fresh. Cheese and meats represented a larger proportion of the diet than I had expected. Whether this has always been the case is hard to tell. Certainly, the mountainous area of Nuoro is a traditional agricultural economy. The philosophy appears to have been to let the animals roam and forage, often in places that were not easily accessible to man. Sardinia is famous for its cheeses made from ewe's milk and goat's milk, particularly the ewe's milk cheese pecorino. Roasted meat from sheep, goat, and wild boar were commonplace. Although we generally consider excessive consumption of meat and cheese to be unhealthy choices, perhaps the naturally organic and free-range nature of the Sardinian versions supports the argument that good-quality food does not harm health. In addition, because the animals live off mountain grasses and other plants, it is likely that both cheese and meat are rich in omega-3 fatty acids—a type of polyunsaturated fat with a number of health benefits (see page 194).

It is also possible that this remote region may have regularly suffered periods of calorie restriction (see page 79) due to seasonal shortages of food.

IS THERE SOMETHING ABOUT SARDINIAN WINES?

The grape varieties found in Sardinia are not so different from those in other parts of the Mediterranean. Cannonau is probably the most popular grape variety for red wines. This is the local name for Grenache or Garnacha, which is widely grown in Spain and southern France; it is also the main grape used in the blend for Châteauneuf-du-Pape in the Rhône Valley. I thought it a good omen for the wines in the Blue Zone that our first visit was to a wine cooperative called Antichi Poderi di Jerzu—Old Farms of Jerzu. Their Cannonau Riserva was called Josto Miglior, after the local doctor who set up this cooperative in 1950. He had lived to the ripe old age of 104. The Jerzu wines are made from grapes grown on some of the oldest vines on the eastern side of the Blue Zone, often at an altitude of 2,300 feet or more.

Another cooperative, the Cantina del Mandrolisai in Sorgono, makes wines from grapes grown on the western side of the Blue Zone. Its red wines are a blend of several grapes: primarily the Sardinian grape Muristellu (also known as Bovale Sardo), together with Cannonau (Grenache), Monica, and Barbera. Tomaso Etzo, the president of the cooperative, was an outstanding host, and he provided a superb lunch accompanied by the cooperative's Rosso Superiore wine. Although we shared a common interest in wine, conversation was slightly hindered by my inability to speak Italian, let alone the local Sardo dialect. There was great amusement at an Englishman visiting Sorgono to investigate the links between wine and longevity. They wanted to have me believe that I was the first Englishman to visit since D. H. Lawrence in 1921, and that because of the large number of centenarians living in the region, they were sure they could introduce me to somebody who remembered him. I was given a copy of the Italian translation of Lawrence's *Sea and Sardinia* describing his trip through the island. A passage had been underlined with pride:

"The Nuoro citizen produced a huge bottle of wine, which he said was *finissimo* . . . So we drank the fine Sorgono wine. It was very good."

I am not sure I tasted the same wine as Lawrence, but I am happy to go along with its description as *finissimo*.

Back in my lab, analyses showed that wines from Nuoro province had higher levels of protective procyanidins than wines from the coastal areas of Sardinia. Although this does not prove the wines are a major factor contributing to longevity in this part of Sardinia, it certainly encouraged me to look at other wine-drinking countries to discover whether the wine being consumed by the longest-lived people was different from wines being drunk elsewhere.

LONGEVITY AND MOUNTAIN LIFESTYLES

Professor Deiana and his colleagues have commented in their reports of the Sardinian centenarians that the majority of "longevity hot spots" around the world are in mountainous regions. Even if life span cannot always be validated, there is a suggestion that living at higher altitude may be linked to longevity.

Studying centenarians in many populations is fraught with problems. The absence of reliable records in isolated locations can make it impossible to validate the claims of long-lived people. And in cultures that venerate the elderly, it is inevitable that ages are often exaggerated. The people of the Caucasus Mountains—which cover parts of Georgia, Armenia, and Azerbaijan—are renowned for their longevity. Stalin was a Georgian, and at one time there was considerable concern in the West over how long he might live. Today in Georgia there are thousands of individuals claiming to be centenarians. In large part this is thought to be due to men assuming the identity of their fathers and grandfathers. In the past this helped them get out of the army, either by avoiding being called up, or enabling them as deserters to escape the authorities. So even if there are a substantial number of centenarians in Georgia, it is impossible to verify their claims. From a wine perspective, this is disappointing because some of the earliest archaeological evidence of wine-making, dating back to about 7000 B.C., has been found in Georgia.

My own studies show that Georgian red wine made from the Saperavi grape has particularly high concentrations of protective procyanidins. Grapes are often grown at altitudes of 1,600 to 4,800 feet. In addition, white wine is often made in a red-wine style, with fermentation of the seeds and skins, to produce an unusual procyanidin-rich white wine called kakhuri. These wines are likely to confer maximum health benefits, so it would not be surprising if there was some genuine longevity among Georgians.

The Hunza Valley in the Himalayas is another location where claims of exceptional longevity have proved impossible to verify. The Hunza are often held up as having a model vegetarian lifestyle. A diet of fruits, fresh vegetables, grains, and walnuts certainly has a flavor of health, and probably an element of calorie restriction (see page 79), but without records the true age of the Hunza "centenarians" remains open to doubt.

A fifteen-year study of Greek villages by researchers from the University of Athens Medical School found a lower number of deaths from heart disease and other causes in a mountain village compared to two lowland areas. This study did not include an analysis of diet or wine consumption.

It is unclear why living in the mountains is protective. One suggestion is that at higher altitude greater energy expenditure during daily tasks and manual work could make a difference in terms of cardiovascular health. Another theory is that air pollution in urban areas is a risk factor for lung and heart disease. Just living in the clean air of the Sardinian or Greek mountains may offer an environment free of the effects of pollution.

WINE AS PART OF THE MEDITERRANEAN DIET

The Greek island of Crete probably has had the greatest influence on dietary advice during the past twenty-five years. This is a consequence of the work of the American nutritionist Ancel Keys, who initiated the Seven Countries Study—and who himself lived to the age of 100. This investigation looked at the relationship between diet and coronary heart disease in the United States, Finland, the Netherlands, Italy, the former Yugoslavia, Greece, and Japan. Between 1958 and 1964, 12,761 men aged forty to fifty-nine years were enrolled in this study. After fifteen years there was clear evidence of a much lower number of deaths in Crete. This correlated with a reduced level of saturated fat and increased level of monounsaturated fat (from olive oil) in the diet. Many nutritionists advocate a "Mediterranean" diet for heart health, but the Cretan version is the classic model for which the strongest supporting evidence is available.

The Cretan diet of the 1960s consisted mainly of fruits and vegetables, breads and grains, beans, nuts, and seeds. Olive oil was the main fat, replacing all other fats and oils. Low to moderate amounts of dairy products such as cheese and yogurt were eaten daily. Eggs were eaten once or twice a week or not at all, and these eggs had a healthier mix of fats than most eggs available today. Fish and poultry were eaten about twice a week. Red meat was eaten only once or twice a month. Processed food was not part of the diet, and foods with added sugar were rarely eaten. However, one feature of this diet that is given little importance, or even ignored completely by nutritionists fearful of advocating alcohol consumption, is that usually one or two glasses of local wine were consumed with meals.

The most important grape varieties for red-wine making in 1960s Crete were Kotsifali and Mandilari. Kotsifali is grown almost uniquely in central Crete, which is the area men were recruited from for the Seven Countries Study. So if the characteristics of any wine had an impact on the findings of the Seven Countries Study, it would have been the local Kotsifali wines. A traditional Cretan blend consisting mainly of Kotsifali, with Mandilari to boost the color and balance the acidity, produces a tannic wine that would not appeal to taste buds attuned to today's fruity, easy-drinking styles. Kotsifali wines can have a leathery mouthfeel when young, which I view as a hallmark of high procyanidin levels. Many Cretan wine producers did not start to bottle their wine until the late 1970s; before that the young wines were sold in bulk, to be drunk within a year of the vintage, so it is likely these contained greater amounts of procyanidins than similar wines today. In the 1970s phylloxera invaded Crete and many vineyards were destroyed. The vineyards have now been replanted, often with the same varieties, but the vines are still comparatively young, and wines made in a more modern style do not necessarily have the same characteristics. However, it is noteworthy that the vines are grown predominantly at an altitude of 1,600 feet or more. Samples of modern Kotsifali-Mandilari blends that I have analyzed show a higher level of procyanidins than typical wines from other countries. These observations suggest that the wine of Crete had more to do with the well-being of people living on this island in the 1960s than is generally given credit.

After twenty-five years of follow-up in the Seven Countries Study, the Cretans had the lowest relative number of deaths from heart disease and all other causes. Forty years after the study started, the Cretans were still doing well: Deaths from coronary heart disease were low and 23 percent were still alive compared to 11 percent in the Netherlands and 16 percent in the U.S.

groups. Apart from age, the main factors that were predictive of mortality were higher than normal blood pressure and smoking.

A number of recent surveys add further support for the Mediterranean diet as a way to maintain optimal health in old age. The results of a ten-year study of 2,339 healthy men and women, aged seventy to ninety years, from eleven European countries, was published in September 2004. Over the study period 935 people died. Calculated as separate factors, those who followed a Mediterranean diet, took daily exercise (equivalent to approximately thirty minutes walking a day), did not smoke, and consumed alcohol regularly had a lower number of deaths. Combining all four lifestyle factors reduced mortality from cancer and heart disease by almost 70 percent. Average alcohol consumption in wine-drinking areas was equivalent to 300 to 400 milliliters (2 to 3 glasses, or about 10 to 13.5 ounces) of wine a day.

Two studies from Greece also give evidence of the benefits of a Mediterranean diet. A study of 22,043 adults found that heart disease and cancer were less common in those sticking strictly to a traditional Mediterranean diet. The second analysis concerned the habits of 489 Greek centenarians. The majority followed a Mediterranean diet. Most of the women did not drink or smoke. Details of the drinking habits of the men have yet to be published.

WINE AND THE REAL FRENCH PARADOX

Many people assume that the French paradox is the idea that red wine consumption accounts for the low occurrence of heart disease in France. In fact, it is the surprising observation that heart disease occurs less often in France than in countries such as the United States and United Kingdom despite similar intakes of saturated fat. Wine consumption has been put forward as a possible explanation for the French paradox, but it is certainly not accepted as the only reason. Having tested wines from a number of places where heart disease is lower and found that they were richer in protective procyanidins, I thought it was time to reexamine whether there was a French paradox that could be explained by wine consumption.

My first step was to see whether there was anywhere in France where there was unusual longevity. I took the view that wines and wine-drinking habits were not uniform across France, so there might be areas where people were living longer because their local wines had special properties such as higher procyanidin levels. I used the 1999 French census data to analyze the regional distribution of men and women aged seventy-five years or more. I focused on values for men because in every study where the details have been published men consume more wine than women, so the benefit of wine is more likely to be observed for men. This analysis identified six regions in southwest and central-southern France where the relative number of men aged seventy-five or older was more than 25 percent higher than the national average (Limousin, Poitou-Charente, Midi-Pyrénées, Languedoc-Roussillon, Aquitaine, Auvergne). In comparison, the region of Alsace had 28 percent fewer men aged seventy-five or older, but it is difficult to ascertain whether this is a residual impact of the two world wars or because it is a mainly white wine drinking area.

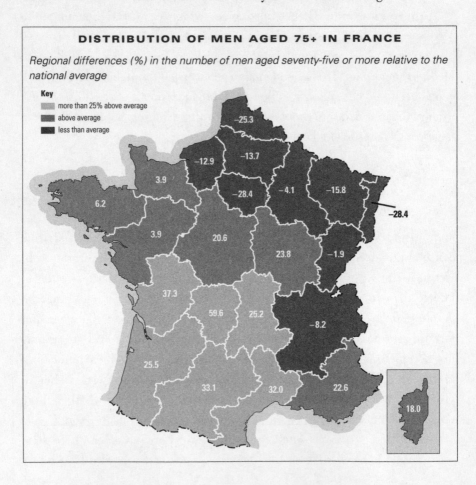

DISTRIBUTION OF MEN AGED 75+ IN FRANCE

Regional differences (%) in the number of men aged seventy-five or more relative to the national average

Key
more than 25% above average
above average
less than average

In order to detect unusual patterns of aging, I needed to analyze these regional data further (each region consists of several départements). To correct for urban migration I identified how many men and women there were aged seventy-five or older in each département. These were then expressed as a ratio. For instance, overall in France, for every man in this age range there are approximately two women aged seventy-five or more (2.12 to be precise). By calculating this ratio for every département I could then look for differences from the average ratio. Only the département of Gers had a ratio of men to women that was more than 20 percent higher than the national average. Gironde, which includes the area of Bordeaux wine production, showed no difference from the national average. Based on the census data, Gers also had double the national average of men aged ninety or more (Gers: 401 per 100,000 people; France overall: 200 per 100,000 people).

So what is special about living in Gers? Is this the home of the real French paradox? Foods high in saturated fat such as foie gras, cassoulet, saucisson,

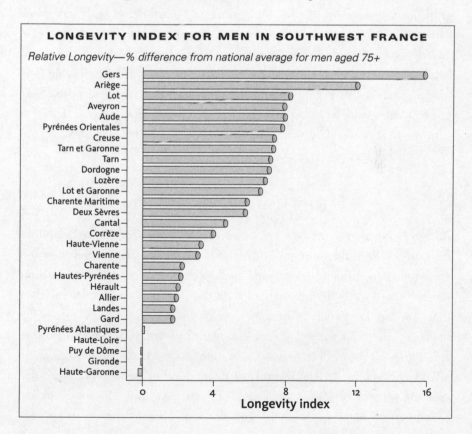

LONGEVITY INDEX FOR MEN IN SOUTHWEST FRANCE

Relative Longevity—% difference from national average for men aged 75+

Gers
Ariège
Lot
Aveyron
Aude
Pyrénées Orientales
Creuse
Tarn et Garonne
Tarn
Dordogne
Lozère
Lot et Garonne
Charente Maritime
Deux Sèvres
Cantal
Corrèze
Haute-Vienne
Vienne
Charente
Hautes-Pyrénées
Hérault
Allier
Landes
Gard
Pyrénées Atlantiques
Haute-Loire
Puy de Dôme
Gironde
Haute-Garonne

0   4   8   12   16
Longevity index

and cheeses are regularly eaten here, so what is the protective factor? Could it be the wine? Is this the French "Red Zone" (the zone of exceptional reds)? Well, after analysis of some wines in my lab, the answer seemed to be a definite yes. If there is anywhere where red wine consumption can explain a local improvement in well-being, it is here. These wines are exceptionally rich in procyanidins. Most red wines do not come near these levels. Madiran, one of the best-known wines of the region, typically contains three to four times more protective procyanidins than my benchmark procyanidin-rich Argentinean Cabernet Sauvignon. Which means that one small glass of this wine can provide more benefit than two bottles of most Australian wine, without the obvious danger of excessive alcohol consumption. So it does seem highly probable that these wines are linked to the survival rate of the men of Gers despite a diet that many cardiologists and dieticians would consider the worst possible choice for heart health.

Why are these wines so special? I think the answer lies in the Tannat grape variety used widely in this region, in combination with traditional winemaking methods. The wines can be astringent, almost brutally tannic, and not at all suitable for casual quaffing. But when sipped with the robust local foods, the high tannins of these wines become hardly noticeable. The winemakers of this region should be encouraged to resist all pressure to move toward modern tastes of berry fruits and soft ripe tannins. Theirs is genuine heart-protecting wine, and this is the real French paradox.

IS WINE THE ELIXIR OF LIFE?

A high proportion of modern red wines could be described as red alcoholic fruit drinks, low in tannins and with little if any health benefit. Because they are so easy to drink without food, many wine drinkers probably consume more of these wines than they should, yet they still may convince themselves that they are doing their heart some good.

Heart disease is the major cause of death in North America and Europe. It is a growing problem in developing nations, as the better-off citizens adopt a Westernized lifestyle. The World Health Organization predicts that heart disease will be responsible for 60 percent of deaths worldwide by 2015. Any key to increased longevity is unlikely to confer much benefit if it doesn't protect the health of the heart and blood vessels. When the Canadian-born physician Sir William Osler wrote in 1862 "a man is only as old as his arteries," he was repeating a commonly accepted expression of his day. Almost 150 years later it still largely holds true. Maintaining vascular health is the key to maintaining overall well-being. Indeed, it is now generally accepted that risk factors for heart disease are also the root cause of many cases of dementia.

So how can we know our vascular age? Until recently it was impossible to gauge with any accuracy while you were still alive. But modern scanning techniques can provide an estimate of your vascular age based on the level of calcium deposited in the walls of your arteries. Readers who have had an EBCT scan (electron-beam computed tomography, also abbreviated to EBT) to assess whether they have coronary heart disease probably will know all about calcium scores. Simply, an EBCT scanner very rapidly takes several X-rays of the heart as a series of slices. From these X-rays it is possible to detect calcium deposits in the walls of the coronary arteries—rather like pipes furring up in areas of hard water—and to provide each individual with a calcium score. Typically calcium scores are graded: no detectable calcium, less than 100, 100 to 400, and higher than 400. The higher the score, the more extensive the level of coronary atherosclerosis, and the greater the likelihood of a coronary event in the future.

The interesting point about vascular aging is that with time everybody has some level of calcium deposits in their coronary arteries. After thousands of people had been scanned by this technique it was clear that calcium scores had a close parallel with age, irrespective of risk factors for heart disease. So somebody aged seventy-five might have a calcium score that is closer to the average for a fifty-year-old, in which case their vascular age could be considered less than their chronological age. Of course, the reverse can also be true.

As far as I know, EBCT scanning has not yet been carried out in any of the hot spots of longevity. Nor has a comparison been undertaken in different wine-drinking areas. However, the Rotterdam Coronary Calcification Study has looked at EBCT coronary calcium scores in people with different drinking habits. Their analysis of calcium scores from 1,795 people, with an average age of seventy, without previous symptoms of coronary heart disease was published in 2004. This provided further evidence that wine reduces coronary heart disease, because people drinking one to two glasses of wine a day were the least likely to have coronary calcium scores over 400. A more detailed analysis of the pattern of calcium scores in wine drinkers might help determine whether wine could be considered an antiaging elixir that slows the speed at which arteries age, and could confirm whether men in some wine regions have arteries that are younger than their years.

TO DRINK OR NOT TO DRINK

The Italian arm of the Seven Countries Study has reported that drinking wine increases life expectancy. The study looked at 1,536 men living in two small villages in northern (Crevalcore) and central (Montegiorgio) Italy. These men were aged forty-five to sixty-four years when they joined the study in 1965 and were followed up for thirty years. The analysis of life expectancy was based on consumption of any alcohol, but 97 percent drank only wine and then it was mostly red. Ignoring whether the men had led physically active lives, those with the highest life expectancy were nonsmokers who consumed four to seven drinks a day (each equivalent to a 4-ounce glass of wine); these drinks were consumed at intervals during the day rather than all at once—a key factor for avoiding the adverse effects normally associated with this level of alcohol consumption. Sedentary men who did not drink or only drank occasionally had the lowest life expectancy—six years less than those drinking a bottle of wine a day. Now, I am not about to claim that not drinking wine can seriously harm your prospects of longevity, but clearly in the context of the lifestyle in these villages it had more positive aspects than negative.

CONCLUSION

Analyses of red wines from several areas of increased longevity led me to conclude that there is a consistent association between such areas and local wines that contain higher levels of procyanidins. This supports the idea that procyanidin-rich red wines make an important contribution to vascular health and long-term well-being. If wine slows vascular aging, it is perhaps more than a coincidence that Methuselah is not only a byword for longevity but also the name for a wine bottle that holds the equivalent of eight normal bottles of wine (i.e., 6 liters or 203 ounces)!

7

THE HUNT FOR PROCYanIDIn-RICH WIneS

Unlike most other diets, *The Red Wine Diet* doesn't tell you to cut out alcohol in order to save a few hundred calories a day. I have already discussed the long-term health benefits of a regular, low-to-moderate intake of alcohol in general and wine in particular. For most adults this is an agreeable and often beneficial approach provided the moderation message is strictly followed. In this chapter I look at the types of wine that are likely to confer the greatest benefit.

Medical research into the health benefits of wine has given a tremendous boost to worldwide sales of red wine in recent years. Often red wine sales have risen in countries and populations where there was no previous tradition of drinking wine. So there are now huge numbers of new wine drinkers who have very different tastes and habits from those found in the long-established winemaking regions. Traditionally, red wine is mainly drunk with food. However, market forces during the past ten to fifteen years, including the tastes of the newly converted red wine drinkers, have created a demand for red wines that are enjoyable to drink at any time. This has led to a completely new style of red wine: fruity and smooth. For some consumers this has been a welcome innovation. However, the demand for this type of wine has changed the way many producers approach their winemaking, and it is this, as I explain below, which may be the cause of a dilemma for wine drinkers.

The head of a large international wine company was reported in 2003 as saying he intended his company to become the Coca-Cola of the winemaking world. For wine lovers this statement rang alarm bells about the direction winemaking is headed: In creating a brand they can market for maximum profit, these large organizations are looking for a wine that is easy to drink in large quantities, bland enough not to challenge the palates of new wine drinkers, and mass produced to taste the same the world over. Among some health professionals it was also seen as a warning about the potential adverse health consequences of this style of wine. It's a shame that the huge international wine conglomerates cannot see beyond short-term profit to a world where their customers lived longer, healthier lives—and could therefore enjoy the products longer! This would be more likely if the wine industry were to support investigations into the specific aspects of red wine that confer health benefits. Winemaking companies claim that their reluctance to support scientific research in this area is due to the likelihood that they will be accused of promoting alcohol consumption. I think it actually comes from a fear of finding that their modern-day products do not match the benefits of many traditionally made wines.

In many ways, the production of red wine is similar to the production of other foods and drinks. New manufacturing methods may result in increased profits but not necessarily in products that are better in terms of overall quality and nutritional benefits, and of course we have no knowledge of the consequences of their long-term consumption over fifty or more years of an individual's life. Yet based on media campaigns and peer pressure we often uncritically swap the new product for the one we have been eating or drinking for years.

The protective effects of red wine on blood vessel health are likely to begin early in life, even if they become fully apparent only years later. Many of the conclusions about the benefits of moderate wine drinking—drawn from studies of men and women aged fifty-five and older—reflect the actions of red wine made using traditional methods. Hence, if there is a major difference in the composition of wines made by current processes and those made using traditional techniques, it will not be surprising if the long-term effects turn out to be markedly different.

Our research has linked some of the important benefits of red wine to procyanidins, which contribute a large part of the astringency of young wines made by traditional methods. But the tannic taste of such wines is precisely what many modern wines lack. From my analyses of wines made in an "easy-drinking" modern style, it seems likely that, in many cases, any health benefit gained from drinking two or three glasses a day of red wine will be substantially reduced if the wine is made in this style. Traditionally made wines have more noticeable tannins, but they also often have a range of fascinating, complex flavors and they complement food far better than many of the bland, sweetish red wines sold today. That said, there are plenty of wines that fall somewhere between the two extremes, and which provide a certain amount of the procyanidins needed to protect our blood vessels.

THE SENSATIONS OF TASTE

Traditional descriptions of taste have four basic characteristics: sweet, sour, bitter, and salty. Anybody who drinks wine regularly will recognize this as a vastly inadequate description of the great variety of flavors that they encounter. In fact, sweet, sour, bitter, and salty are just points of reference across a whole spectrum of taste sensations. Work undertaken by the Human Genome Project indicates that there are fifty to hundred genes for different taste receptors. Each receptor binds specific chemicals—much like a lock and key. When a chemical comes along that fits well, it binds to the receptor, which then sends signals to the brain, where the taste information is processed.

Beyond the basic taste sensations on the tongue, our sense of smell registers volatile elements on odor receptors in our nasal cavity. The tongue and the nose send signals to the brain, and it is the combination of a set of chemicals (sometimes thousands of different molecules) that the brain interprets as being responsible for a particular taste. These are the flavors named by wine writers: black currant, raspberry, cedar, chocolate, and so on.

Scientists now recognize the existence of a fifth taste sensation—umami (Japanese for "delicious"). Umami is the savory taste of glutamate (an amino acid, one of the building blocks of most proteins), and it has its own taste receptor. Most people are familiar with the flavor enhancer monosodium glutamate: It is added to some Japanese and Chinese food and to many ready-made soups, pâtés, pies, and other meat products; glutamate is also present in foods such as salt-cured and fermented products and some cheeses.

ACQUIRED TASTES

Individual variation in taste sensations may be very marked; Some people always add three spoonfuls of sugar to their coffee, which would make it undrinkably sweet to others. And the flavors in a particular wine appreciated by one person may not give the same pleasure to his or her companions. This can be attributed partly to genetic differences and partly to learned or acquired tastes.

Children often favor sweet foods, but this bias usually diminishes in adulthood. Similarly, young palates seem to dislike bitterness. When I was an inquisitive little boy my father would let me sip his home-brewed beer—yuck! But by the age of sixteen I had completely lost my aversion to bitter hop flavors. This adaptation of taste is a well-recognized phenomenon. Children are often given watered-down wine in France and Italy, where regular moderate wine consumption is seen as a natural part of any meal.

Another aspect of taste adaptation occurs when exposure to bitter substances heightens the sensitivity to sugar or sweetness; tannic wines may reduce the desire for sweet foods. Salty foods seem to intensify bitter and sour flavors. So a salt-rich diet may cause aversion to tannic wines; the excess salt in many of today's foods may go some way to accounting for the popularity of soft, fruity alcoholic drinks—including many mass-produced red wines.

Acidity provides the refreshing element to fruit, be it a crisp apple, a lemon, or a juicy grape. Acidity enhances the sensation of sweetness. All wines need acidity—without it they taste dull and flabby—and an experienced winemaker uses his or her skill to ensure that there is neither too much nor too little acidity, but just enough to balance the elements of fruit and tannin and create a harmonious whole.

Wine and food pairing is an art that many wine drinkers learn through trial and error, and it is certainly true that different food flavors affect the perceived taste of wine. Red meat and game, especially when cooked rare, can soften the astringency of tannin. The savory umami taste of certain protein-rich foods, including some cheeses, can make some wines taste stronger and more tannic; that is why sweet white wines or port are often better accompaniments to cheese than red wine. Similarly, highly spiced Indian and Thai food can turn some wines into unpleasant beasts. Many wine writers recommend fruity (unoaked) white wines and low-tannin reds for spicy curries; I usually drink beer. Has the increased popularity of spicy and salty food fueled the global trend for soft, fruity, low-tannin red wines?

Taste adaptation may be part of changing both your wine drinking and other dietary habits to achieve a healthier balance. Tannic wines may reduce the craving for sweet foods and drinks; from a health point of view, this can only be a good thing. Tannic wines are almost always best with food, which is the best way to include wine as part of a healthy lifestyle. In this chapter I hope to inspire you to try some different wines—perhaps more tannic than you may be used to—until you find a selection that you truly enjoy.

THE TASTE OF POLYPHENOLS

Polyphenols are a diverse group of chemicals (see page 33) that are relatively unstable, spontaneously undergoing chemical reactions to form more complex

THE ACID TEST

The way acidity affects taste can be tested in a simple experiment: Make a cup of fairly strong tea using a traditional English tea (i.e. a black tea, sometimes called English breakfast tea), do not add any milk or sugar, and allow it to cool until you can drink a mouthful or two. Then squeeze a quarter of a lemon into the tea, stir well, and taste again. You should notice that the tannic and bitter tastes of the tea are substantially reduced. The tea also becomes slightly lighter in color (more easily seen if you are using a white cup), which shows that the acidity of the lemon has modified chemically the tea tannins; these changes, together with the effect of acidity on your taste receptors, makes this tea easier to drink without sugar or milk. In a similar way, tannic wines with good levels of acidity are much more palatable than tannic wines with low acidity.

molecules, and are vulnerable to oxidation and further modification over time. The huge spectrum of different tastes in wine can be attributed in large part to the variety of polyphenols wine contains. Polyphenols also interact with acidity to create additional flavor sensations. In winemaking the main source of polyphenols is the grapes, but aging in oak introduces additional polyphenols that add to the complexity of the wine.

Some of the most abundant polyphenols in young red wines are procyanidins. Young wines are often astringent, and procyanidins are thought to be a major contributor to astringency. This is a mouthfeel that is not classified as a standard taste sensation (although it is sometimes confused with bitterness). Astringency is sensed as a rough or dry mouthfeel, often referred to as mouth-puckering. It is caused by polyphenols in the wine interacting with salivary proteins. This interaction causes the polyphenols to precipitate and become insoluble so that the lubricant effect of saliva is temporarily lost. Acidity has the opposite effect: It makes your mouth water. Wines with nothing to recommend them but their astringency are unlikely to be much fun, unless the astringency is balanced by acidity.

The precise molecules that cause astringency are not yet fully understood. Traditional cider, for instance, is rich in procyanidins but generally not mouth-puckering. The most mouth-puckering thing I have ever tasted is an unripe kaki fruit, and these fruit have other tannins besides procyanidins. Strong tea is also tannic and astringent but not particularly rich in beneficial procyanidins. So I think the mouth-drying sensation of some young wines is most likely due to the combined effects of procyanidins with other polyphenol components.

Astringency declines as wines age and polyphenols polymerize into more complex chemicals, condensed tannins, which form a sediment at the bottom of the bottle.

OAK TANNINS

Oak tannins are in many ways more appealing to taste than grape tannins because they do not have the same astringency. However, oak tannins—the gallotannins from the wood itself—do not have much biological activity and do not have the same protective effects on blood vessel function as procyanidins.

Aging wines in oak can increase the sensation of tannins in the final product, although much of the oaky flavor is actually derived from the charring of the inside of the wooden barrels, which is part of the process of barrel making. New oak barrels give more oak flavor than older ones. Mass-produced wines often have oak chips added—during a period of storage in stainless steel tanks—to create a similar flavor to wine aged in oak barrels in the traditional way.

LOOKING FOR CLUES

Many wine drinkers are overawed by the number of wines they are faced with in stores, online, and on restaurant menus. Quotes and comments from wine writers are useful only if you know and trust the taste of the writer in question. The marketing-speak on the label is often quite meaningless. The wines that, to a casual reader, sound most seductive—"easy drinking, soft, smooth"—are often dull and lacking in the acidity, tannins, and complexity that make for an interesting drink. Their soft, fruity smoothness may also disguise the fact that many of them contain more than 14 percent alcohol, so drinkers are often consuming too much alcohol, even as they miss out on the protective effects they seek.

"Concentrated fruit flavors, with great acidity and a fine, full tannic finish; good aging potential." These are the type of tasting notes that, in combination, suggest a promising wine. Instead of easy drinking, we should be looking for a more challenging wine that can be sipped and enjoyed with food but not knocked back in vast quantity.

LEARNING FROM THE LABEL

Just as regulations in many countries require the alcohol content of wine to be printed on the label, I see no reason why in the future it should not be a legal requirement to include a statement of the procyanidin content. International criteria will need to be set, as different laboratories currently have different ways of measuring procyanidins, but I predict that sooner or later we will be told exactly which health benefits we can expect from a glass of wine.

The protective effect of certain polyphenols is not confined to wine (see Chapter 4). Food and drink companies around the world are interested in the whole area of polyphenols, and from my position as a research scientist I know that it will not be long before you are all hearing more about the health benefits of these molecules. Functional foods and supplements will appear on the market, some potentially beneficial, others useless. One of my aims in writing this book is to help you learn the optimum daily dose of procyanidins for maximum health benefit: 300 to 500 milligrams of procyanidins is an ideal target to aim for. More might be better—but remember this should be from a variety of sources, not just wine!

PROCYANIDIN-RICH RED WINES: THE KEY INFLUENCES

The factors affecting the amount of procyanidins in wine can be divided broadly into three areas: vineyard environment, the grape, and the winemaker. The consumer can also influence the amount of procyanidins by choosing whether to drink a wine young or only after storing or cellaring for several years—over time, the procyanidin content of any wine will gradually reduce.

There is a complex interaction in the vineyard between the type of soil, the amount of rainfall or irrigation, and the sunlight and temperature. Some of these factors are beyond the winegrower's control and account for vintage variation.

KEY FACTORS IN THE VINEYARD FOR MAKING WINES WITH HIGH PROCYANIDIN CONTENT

- *Infertile land*
- *Well-established vines*
- *Long, slow ripening*
- *High altitudes*
- *Low yields*

- Land that is infertile or otherwise unsuitable for other agricultural purposes is often ideal for vineyards. Many of the world's best traditional wines are grown on mixtures of chalk and clay, gravel over limestone, slate, or steep rocky slopes.

- Established vines generally do not need much water because their roots reach deep into the soil; irrigation may increase the amount of wine you can make, but it also dilutes it. Excess water from irrigation or too much rain at the wrong time of year also encourages excessive leaf growth, which prevents ripening.

- Slow ripening tends to boost the levels of all polyphenols. In classic cool-climate regions, the ideal long ripening season has warm to hot sunny days and cool nights. In hotter parts of the world, a longer season may be achieved by planting vineyards at higher altitudes or in valleys subject to sea breezes or fog.

- Two key enzymes involved in polyphenol synthesis are increased by ultraviolet (UV) light. So grapes grown at higher altitudes, where there is more UV exposure, potentially could achieve higher levels of procyanidins.

- Increased exposure of grapes to direct sunlight during ripening stimulates polyphenol synthesis. But if the grapes get too hot, polyphenol synthesis is suppressed. Under very hot conditions the acidity of the grape juice also drops. Hence, canopy management (the various techniques of vine trellising and pruning, which determine how much sunlight reaches the grapes) can have a profound effect on grape polyphenol composition, which in turn alters the flavor characteristics of the wine.

- Reducing yield by removing bunches of grapes ("green harvest") before ripening can increase the quality of the grapes that are left and give a more concentrated wine.

- Low-yielding vines generally give the best quality wines. Yields tend to reduce naturally after the vines are twenty to thirty years old, so for economic reasons some growers uproot and replace the vines, but others treasure and make a sales feature of their old vines, which can live for more than 100 years.

I have noticed that wines made from old vines often have a higher procyanidin level than wines made from younger vines from the same winery. I don't know whether this reflects a genuine difference in the quality of the fruit coming from older vines or whether it is influenced by vineyard management and winemaking techniques. The grapes from older vines are frequently used to make a winery's top wine, so more care may be taken with these vines at every stage.

Grape variety can make a big difference to the procyanidin content of wine—but only if vineyard management and the winemaker exploit the advantage that a particular variety provides. The smaller the grape and the greater the number of seeds per berry, the higher the potential amounts of procyanidins.

In my experience the grape yielding the most procyanidin-rich wines is Tannat, one of the traditional grapes of southwest France. Cabernet Sauvignon also has small berries and a high ratio of seed to pulp, and when I compared Cabernet Sauvignon with Malbec wines grown in similar conditions in Argentina, the Cabernets tended to have more procyanidins. So grape variety may be more of an influence than some other aspects.

Although Malbec lost out to Cabernet in a direct comparison, I have had very good results from several Malbec-based wines, both those grown in high-altitude vineyards in Argentina and those from Malbec's traditional homeland of Cahors in southwest France.

My most recent analysis of a selection of red wines was designed to follow up some of the clues I unearthed while writing this book. Italian wines, for example, are known as excellent partners to food, with a touch of bitterness and good acidity balanced with tannins. Among others, I was impressed by Nebbiolo—one of the classic grapes of northwest Italy, Sangiovese—the grape of Chianti and a number of other Tuscan wines, and Aglianico, an ancient grape variety grown in southern Italy. It is difficult to generalize about grape varieties because the influence of the winemaker is crucial (see the following page).

Although differences in the amount of procyanidins in red wine clearly occur because of the grape variety and the vineyard environment, the winemaker holds the key to what ends up in the bottle. The most important aspect of the winemaking process for ensuring high procyanidins in red wines is the contact time between the liquid and the grape seeds and skins. Procyanidins start to be extracted from the seeds during fermentation when the alcohol concentration reaches about 6 percent. Depending on the fermentation temperature, it may be two to three days or more before this extraction process starts. Grape skins float and seeds sink, so the number of times they are pushed down and stirred into the fermenting wine also increases extraction of procyanidins. Even so, extraction is a slow process and, after fermentation is complete, many red wines are left to macerate with their seeds and skins for days or even weeks in order to extract all the color, flavor, and tannins. Wines that have a contact time of less than seven days will have a relatively low level of procyanidins. Wines with a contact time of ten to fourteen days have decent levels, and those with contact times of three weeks or more have the highest. Good merchants know which wines are made this way—so do ask!

When making many lighter-style wines, the fermenting juice is separated from the grape seeds and skins before the procyanidins have been extracted. Because of the lack of tannins and other extracted polyphenols, these wines have less structure and will not have the same ability to evolve into something more interesting over time—they are not intended to be kept for long periods. This style of wine cannot offer the consumer maximum health benefit.

To make the wine clear, to make it microbiologically stable, and to reduce harsh tannins, wine may be fined and/or filtered. Fining is a traditional process, and most wines undergo some degree of fining. Fining agents, such as gelatin, isinglass, egg white, bentonite, or a chemical called polyvinylpolypyrrolidone (PVPP), are added to the fermented wine to remove microscopic solid particles. The fining agent binds with a variety of wine polyphenols, including procyanidins, then settles out and can be easily removed. Filtration requires investment in expensive equipment, but it is a quick and efficient way to ensure clear and consistent wine. Depending on the degree of fining or filtration, and on the substances used, the amount of procyanidins in a wine may be substantially reduced.

Wine will eventually "fall bright," or clear itself, but this requires time and careful racking off of the clear liquid from the solids that have fallen to the bottom of the barrel. Whenever possible, choose wines that have not been fined or filtered but allowed to settle naturally; these wines may eventually develop a small but harmless deposit in the bottle.

Deciding how long to keep a wine before you drink it can influence the amount of procyanidins that are left. This is because procyanidins are relatively unstable molecules that over time form condensed tannins, which appear as a dark reddish-brown sediment at the bottom of the bottle. Long aging is probably not in your best interests from a health point of view; neither will it do much for the taste of inexpensive everyday wines. Communities known for their longevity or exceptional good health, such as those in Crete, southwest France, and Sardinia, traditionally would drink their local wines young—usually no more than three years after the vintage— often drawing them straight from the barrel; this certainly would contribute to a high level of procyanidins in the wine.

The decrease in procyanidins is a gradual process; if a wine has a high level of procyanidins when it is first made, it still will have good levels at five years old. But differences are likely to be greater after ten years, depending on cellaring conditions (particularly temperature) and the overall structure of the wine.

THE HUNT FOR PROCYANIDIN-RICH WINES

When I first started wine research I hoped I might be able to demonstrate that inexpensive wines were just as good as higher-priced ones in terms of potential health benefit. Once I realized that it was traditional long fermentation and maceration of grape seeds and skins in the juice that made the most procyanidin-rich wines, I saw that I might be promoting a style of winemaking I have seen described on French wine labels as *vinifié à*

NOT WHAT THE DOCTOR ORDERED

The chemical fining agent polyvinylpolypyrrolidone (PVPP) is sometimes used to clarify wine; it is also often used in tablet-making to provide an inert matrix (a chemically unreactive substance in which the drug is incorporated), and is found in pharmaceutical products such as tablets and some dietary supplements. Its presence is rarely if ever indicated, yet it binds all polyphenols so strongly that taking such a tablet at the same time as a polyphenol-rich food or drink will completely prevent absorption of polyphenols such as procyanidins. So the warning not to drink alcohol when taking some medicines can be seen in a different light: the medication might neutralize the benefits from the polyphenols in red wine! But please do not stop taking your medications.

l'ancienne sans compromis—winemaking the old-fashioned way, without any concessions to the demands of modern tastes.

However, as I continue to taste and analyze more wines I realize the situation is not black and white, old versus new. Many winemakers combine long fermentation and maceration with a variety of modern techniques to improve fruit characteristics and overall quality. Their wines retain decent amounts of procyanidins. I am sure such wines will become increasingly popular as consumers recognize how well they go with food.

Although currently wines are not analyzed routinely for their procyanidin content, there is a fairly simple test to measure the total polyphenol content, or phenolic index, which includes tannins, procyanidins, anthocyanins (which provide the grapes' color), and other polyphenols. Winemakers are increasingly quoting IPT (from the French, (Index of Total Polyphenlos) in their technical data, which can often be found on the Internet and in wine magazines. In general, the higher the IPT, the greater the amount of procyanidins in a wine.

However, I must be honest and tell you that IPT measures quantity of polyphenols, not quality. Some grapes, for example Syrah and Malbec, have high IPT scores because of their high anthocyanin content. This is not to say that you won't find examples of wines made from Syrah and Malbec with perfectly good procyanidin levels, but from my own laboratory work I can say that, other things being equal, Cabernet Sauvignon is likely to have higher procyanidin levels than most other "international" grape varieties.

RECOMMENDING RED WINES

My research has shown that in areas of increased longevity the red wines being drunk on a daily basis are much richer in procyanidins than the average wine. After analysis, I have created a rating on a scale of ❤ to ❤❤❤❤❤, where most red wines achieve at least a ❤ rating. Even white wines have some health benefit, because they increase HDL-cholesterol (the good form of cholesterol; see Chapter 2), so ❤ represents the bottom of the range for red wines. Even so, I have occasionally found red wines that are below the level I would consider giving a ❤ rating. The ❤❤❤❤❤ rating represents the best wines I have found.

♥ = average
♥♥ = shows promise
♥♥♥ = good
♥♥♥♥ = very good
♥♥♥♥♥ = excellent

A 4-ounce glass of super-rich ♥♥♥♥♥ wine typically contains at least 120 milligrams procyanidins, and often more; a glass of procyanidin-rich ♥♥♥ wine typically will provide 60 to 90 milligrams of procyanidins; an average ♥ wine may contain 30 to 45 milligrams of procyanidins; the ♥♥ and ♥♥♥♥ ratings are intermediate levels—better than the rating below but not reaching the one above.

One important advantage of choosing wines with high procyanidin levels is that less needs to be consumed to achieve the optimal benefit. One glass of ♥♥♥♥♥ wine or two glasses of ♥♥♥ wine typically will provide the same amount of procyanidins as three to four glasses of an average wine.

The very best results I've had in my laboratory have been from Madiran wines (read more about them on pages 114–17). These wines have some of the highest procyanidin levels I've encountered, as a result of the local grape variety, Tannat, and the traditional long fermentation and maceration. Long fermentation and maceration are important wherever wine is made, and from other parts of the world I have had good results from wines made from grapes grown at high altitude and/or from old or low-yielding vines.

The basic, mass-produced, branded wines sold in many wine bars and pubs generally don't conform to the above criteria and, when analyzed, have disappointingly low levels of procyanidins. They are also often deceptively high in alcohol. I believe that the types of wine that are best for health are those designed to be sipped as an accompaniment to food, not those made for casual quaffing. If you're thirsty, drink water!

With many thousands of wines being made around the world each year, and with so many variables in climate, growing conditions, grape varieties, and blends, a dedicated laboratory would be needed to analyze wines systematically. The wine from one vintage does not guarantee that earlier or later vintages are comparable. I can't give you enough examples to cover what you might want to drink every day, but this chapter should give you a good idea of the types of wines that are likely to be most beneficial, with some useful specific examples. What follows is a personal look at some of the red wines I have analyzed and enjoyed—and rated as good to excellent in terms of their procyanidin content.

ARGENTINA

Here's a country that has all the right conditions—including some very high-altitude vineyards—but a profusion of wines made for quaffing means that Argentinian wines don't all perform equally well on the procyanidin front. Malbec, one of Argentina's distinctive grape varieties, is rich in tannins and damsony flavor: when made from old, low-yielding vines in a traditional style, with long fermentation and maceration, it is likely to have good ♥♥♥ procyanidin levels. I've recently analyzed a ♥♥♥♥♥ Malbec Reserva from Altos Las Hormigas; this wine undergoes four weeks of fermentation and maceration. However, a mass-produced Malbec may rate only ♥ or ♥♥.

Bodega Catena Zapata is one of Argentina's best-known wineries, with vineyards at altitudes between 2,600 and 5,000 feet. All aspects of vineyard management are carefully controlled, and yields are kept low. I have analyzed

---

FINDING MORE INFORMATION

The most procyanidin-rich wines are generally those where the grapes (seeds, skins, and all) have remained in contact with the wine during fermentation and afterward, for a period of maceration. This sort of technical information is seldom seen on wine bottles. In the future, procyanidin content may appear on the label as routinely as alcohol content, but until then, you can be proactive about finding more information. Many wineries include technical information about their winemaking techniques on their Web sites; look for a contact time of at least ten days for a good level of procyanidins. A good wine merchant should be able to provide information on how their wines are made, so ask if you are uncertain.

several vintages of Cabernet Sauvignon in both the Catena and Catena Alta ranges and rated them ♥♥♥, verging on ♥♥♥♥.

Bodega Norton was established in 1895 and its top wine, Norton Privada, is one I never fail to enjoy. It is a blend of Malbec, Cabernet Sauvignon, and Merlot, from vines that are fifty to eighty years old and grown at altitudes between 2,800 and 3,600 feet. They are fermented for seven days and left to macerate for an additional twenty-five to thirty days. Analysis has shown a consistent ♥♥♥ rating.

AUSTRALIA

I'm very sorry to tell you that the big brands that have led the huge expansion of Australian wine exports are, on the whole, low in procyanidins. Wine critics also notice that these wines have been getting sweeter in order to appeal to the taste of the U.S. mass market. However, don't despair, because there are many wines made by independent wineries in Australia—particularly from Cabernet Sauvignon—that do deliver the goods. Look for wines from smaller, often family-owned companies, which draw on the best aspects of traditional methods. If the back label mentions old vines, low yields, and long contact (fermentation and maceration) times, so much the better.

South of Adelaide, the sunny, maritime McLaren Vale is home to many wineries and boasts a number of low-yielding old vineyards. A favorite producer of mine here is D'Arenberg: Their High Trellis Cabernet Sauvignon has a good ♥♥♥ procyanidin rating. Farther south still, the Coonawarra region is known for its Cabernet Sauvignon wines, grown in limestone, with a thin layer of rich red topsoil. One of the biggest and best producers here is Wynns, whose Cabernet Sauvignon ♥♥♥ contains good levels of procyanidins. Balnaves of Coonawarra, a small, family-owned company, produces a promising ♥♥ Cabernet Sauvignon that narrowly missed out on ♥♥♥.

The Barossa Valley, also in South Australia, is also renowned for its low-yielding and very old vines, particularly Shiraz and Grenache; somewhat surprisingly, I have not been able to find many procyanidin-rich examples.

CHILE

With plenty of old established vineyards, there is no reason why a good number of Chilean wines—especially Cabernet Sauvignon made with long fermentation and maceration—should not have good procyanidin levels. Benchmark ♥♥♥ Cabernet Sauvignons I have tasted include Concha y Toro's Casillero del Diablo, Cono Sur Reserve, Errazuriz, Montes, and Montes Alpha, Valdivieso Reserve, and Veramonte.

FRANCE

BORDEAUX   There are thousands of châteaux in Bordeaux, from Classed Growths to mass-market brands. I have not had the opportunity to test the stratospherically priced Classed Growths, but based on laboratory evidence that suggests that long extraction times account for a high level of beneficial procyanidins, it seems likely that there will be many heart-friendly wines at the top end of the market, where long maceration is the norm. However, I have analyzed enough modestly priced red Bordeaux to be able to say that large numbers of them have better-than-average procyanidin levels (between ♥♥ and ♥♥♥). Some may be even higher in procyanidins: I recently found a ♥♥♥♥ wine, Château Montaiguillon, from the lowly appellation of Montagne St. Émilion—and this was from the difficult 2002 vintage.

Most of Bordeaux's red wines are made from a promising blend of grapes, predominantly Cabernet Sauvignon, Merlot, and Cabernet Franc in varying proportions, but vintages and winemaking styles are prone to enormous variation. One reason they may not rate more highly overall is that many Bordeaux wines are fined with egg whites (see page 103), which reduces procyanidin levels. This is one region where you really need to be proactive in finding out about individual wines (from Web sites or in-depth wine guides).

BURGUNDY   Pinot Noir, the grape that makes red Burgundy, generally is not high in procyanidins, but wines from the village of Pommard have a reputation for being unusually tannic and long-lived. The soil here is high in both limestone and clay, and the interaction between these soils may account for the sturdiness of the wines. My analyses have found Pommard wines with ratings between ♥♥♥ and ♥♥♥♥♥.

SOUTHWEST   My research into longevity led me to discover the exciting properties of the ♥♥♥♥♥ wines of Madiran, based on the Tannat grape, which I discuss in more detail on pages 114 to 117. Cahors wines, traditionally known for being dark, almost black, tannic, and ideal with food, are based on Malbec (also known as Auxerrois) and when well made, with long maceration times, can be high in procyanidins. Clos Triguedina, Château de Gaudou Cuvée Tradition, and Château du Cèdre Cuvée le Cèdre are all ♥♥♥♥ Cahors wines.

LANGUEDOC-ROUSSILLON   It is impossible to generalize about this vast area. Quality-focused producers have planted Cabernet Sauvignon and Merlot alongside the traditional—and sometimes very old—Carignan, Grenache, Syrah, and Mourvèdre. I've particularly enjoyed the following wines: Domaine de l'Hortus Grande Cuvée ♥♥♥, from Pic St. Loup; Côtes du Roussillon-Villages wines made by Domaine des Chênes (Le Mascarou ♥♥♥), Vignerons Catalans (Cuvée Extrême ♥♥♥), and Les Maîtres Vignerons de Tautavel ♥♥♥; Gérard Bertrand's Corbières Boutenac Domaine de Villemajou ♥♥♥; Vignoble du Loup Blanc's La Mère Grand ♥♥♥♥♥, and Domaine Tour Trencavel's Lo Cagarol ♥♥♥♥ from Minervois, plus, from the superior zone of Minervois la Livinière, Domaine la Rouvioule ♥♥♥♥♥, Les Trois Blason's Cuvée Gaïa ♥♥♥♥, and Gérard Bertrand's Château Laville Bertrou ♥♥♥. One of the most famous wines of the south of France is the tannic yet rich Cabernet Sauvignon–based Mas de Daumas Gassac. The exceptional 2003 vintage produced an impressive ♥♥♥♥♥ wine, while the lighter 2004 vintage achieved ♥♥♥.

RHÔNE   The Rhône Valley has two distinct zones: the cooler north, where red wines are made from 100 percent Syrah grapes, and the warmer south, where Grenache and other grapes join Syrah in the blends for Châteauneuf-du-Pape, Côtes du Rhône, and others. All are highly compatible with food. From the Cave de Tain cooperative in the north I've enjoyed Cornas "Arènes Sauvages" ♥♥♥♥ and Hermitage ♥♥♥: The good ratings may be due to a combination of factors—soil (granitic sand), old vines, low yields, and long maceration times. In the south I've had inconsistent results from wines made from old-vines Grenache. On the other hand, some inexpensive Côtes du Rhône reds have done well in laboratory analyses: Domaine Chapoton ♥♥♥; Domaine Ferraton ♥♥♥.

ITALY

NORTH Piedmont's most famous grape is the highly acidic, deeply tannic Nebbiolo, which ripens late in the autumn. Barolo and Barbaresco are the best known, usually 100 percent Nebbiolo wines, and traditionally have long maceration times of three or four weeks. Among the Nebbiolo wines I have rated most highly are Ciabot-Berton's Barolo ♥♥♥♥, Langhe Nebbiolo De Forville ♥♥♥♥, and Pio Cesare's Barolo ♥♥♥. Nebbiolo is not the only exciting grape in this region; I have been equally impressed by Dolcetto and Barbera: Luigi Einaudi's Dolcetto di Dogliani ♥♥♥♥, Vajra's Dolcetto d'Alba ♥♥♥, and Ca' del Matt's Barbera d'Asti Terre Caude ♥♥♥.

The Veneto region of northeastern Italy is best known for light, cherryish Valpolicella, but I'd like to draw attention to the wines of an exceptional producer, Allegrini: Palazzo della Torre ♥♥♥♥ and La Grola ♥♥♥.

CENTER Tuscany's Sangiovese is the most widely planted grape in Italy and is the main grape used in Chianti. However, there are so many different winemaking styles, Sangiovese clones, and alternative names for the grape, that any generalization is next to impossible. Nevertheless, I have had some very good tastings of Sangiovese-based wines, including Avignonesi's Vino Nobile di Montepulciano ♥♥♥, Isole e Olena's Chianti Classico ♥♥♥, Cantine Leonardo's Chianti ♥♥♥, and II Colombaio di Cencio's Chianti Classico Riserva ♥♥♥. Morellino di Scansano, one of Sangiovese's alter egos, proved excellent, with both Le Pupille and Lohsa achieving ♥♥♥♥.

I was also pleasantly surprised by Luigi D'Alessandro's II Bosco, a Tuscan Syrah that rated ♥♥♥, and Poggio Bestiale ♥♥♥♥, a Bordeaux-style blend of Cabernet Sauvignon, Merlot, and Cabernet Franc made by Fattoria di Magliano in the Maremma area on the southern coast of Tuscany.

Umbria, Tuscany's neighbor, makes Sangiovese-based wines and international-style reds (Sportoletti's Villa Fidelia, a Merlot-Cabernet blend, rates ♥♥♥), but its specialty is the tannic Sagrantino grape. Arnaldo-Caprai's Sagrantino di Montefalco Collepiano ♥♥♥♥♥ is not only rich and powerful; it also has one of the highest procyanidin contents I've ever found.

SOUTHERN ITALY, SICILY, SARDINIA The ancient, late-ripening Aglianico grape keeps its acidity well in southern Italy's hot climates. Outstanding among those I've tried are Di Majo Norante's Aglianico Contado ♥♥♥♥ and Vesevo's Beneventano Aglianico ♥♥♥♥.

Sicily's top grape is the dark, highly acidic Nero d'Avola, and in the right hands it can produce wines that are both delicious and beneficial. It's often blended with other grapes: with Syrah in Alire's Fatascia ♥♥♥♥ and with Cabernet Sauvignon and Merlot in Ceuso ♥♥♥♥.

Sardinia was the base for much of my research into longevity. The Cantina del Mandrolisai, where local grape varieties grow in high-altitude vineyards, produces the traditional, procyanidin-rich Rosso Superiore del Mandrolisai ♥♥♥♥♥ and the newer Kent'annos (which means "one hundred years") ♥♥♥♥. A number of other Sardinian wines rated ♥♥♥.

PORTUGaL

The steep granite slopes of the Douro in northern Portugal are increasingly producing good red wines that make great partners for hearty food. They're made from a blend of grapes, one of the most promising being Touriga Nacional. Recently I've enjoyed one from Quinta do Crasto ♥♥♥ and another from Quinta de Fafide ♥♥♥♥.

spain

Rioja, Spain's most famous red wine, comes from a large area, in a variety of styles. Basic mass-produced wines are least likely to be beneficial, along with Gran Reservas, which are aged for many years before they go on sale and thus are well on their way to losing many of their procyanidins. One of my recent favorites was made by the high-profile producer Telmo Rodriguez, who tends to use older vines; I rated it ❤❤❤. The dark reds of Ribera del Duero are, like Rioja, often based on the Tempranillo grape, sometimes with Cabernet Sauvignon and Merlot in the blend. I was pleasantly surprised by the Ribera del Duero Reserva under the Altos de Tamaron label, which I rated ❤❤❤❤.

URUGUAY

Uruguay is one of the few places in the world outside southwest France that grows a substantial proportion of the procyanidin-rich Tannat grape. However, Uruguayan Tannats seem to be made in a lighter style and few of them compare to Madiran for procyanidin content. One exception I have found is Catamayor Tannat ❤❤❤❤ made by Bodegas Castillo Viejo.

UNITED STATES

Wine production is concentrated in the Pacific Coast states. Grapes are grown almost anywhere that climatic conditions, and land prices, permit, and there is no doubt that key geographical and environmental factors have a significant impact on both overall quality and on procyanidin content. One practice that I consider counterproductive, yet is increasingly common, is the use of extended hang times, where ripe grapes are left on the vine longer to produce smoother wines. This leads to overripe grapes with lower amounts of procyanidins, and because sugars are more concentrated the resulting alcohol levels are higher—exceeding 16 percent for some wines—so on both counts wines made in this way are not ideal. However, U.S. wineries often provide very detailed information—read the technical/winemaker's notes to discover whether the grapes' contact (fermentation and maceration) time was at least ten to fourteen days, and look for wines described as having firm tannins.

CALIFORNIA Cabernet Sauvignon is the grape of choice for classic California reds, and it has given me the best results: ❤❤❤❤ for Robert

Mondavi Napa Valley Reserve and ❤❤❤ for Mondavi's regular Napa Valley and Private Selection Cabernets. Other ❤❤❤ Cabernets include Franciscan Oakville Estate, Hess Select, and Mount Veeder Winery. Promising ❤❤ wines can be found in all sectors of the market, from Ridge Monte Bello (at the top end of the price range), to Beringer (somewhere in the middle), to budget-priced Gallo Turning Leaf. I've also had some good results from Cabernet wines from higher altitude vineyards in the cooler northern part of the state. Zinfandels look promising, though not outstanding, with ❤❤ for both the Old Vine Zinfandel and Vintners' Blend from Ravenswood.

WASHINGTON STATE   Long summer days and cool nights in the Columbia Valley, where most of the state's grapes are grown, result in deeply colored, intensely flavored wines. I gave my highest ratings to two Bordeaux-style blends from Matthews Cellars: Red ❤❤❤❤❤ and Claret ❤❤❤❤. Gordon Brothers' Cabernet Sauvignon and three Cabernets from Woodward Canyon—Nelms Road, Old Vines, and Artist Series—also rated ❤❤❤❤. I have enjoyed ❤❤❤ Cabernets from Amavi, Chateau Sainte Michelle, Columbia Crest (Grand Estates), L'Ecole No. 41, and Pepper Bridge. Pendulum Red, a blend of eight grapes, also rated ❤❤❤.

THE REAL FRENCH PARADOX

The French paradox—low levels of heart disease in France despite high saturated fat consumption—has intrigued wine drinkers since it was first reported. The question I asked was whether French wines were universally good for heart health or was the effect restricted to certain areas of France. As revealed in Chapter 6, my research led me to analyze the wines in the Gers area of southwest France. If there was truly a French paradox, then it was here. Gers had double the national average of men aged ninety or more. If red wine is the protecting force, then this region's wines must be providing special benefits. Now, I'm a fairly skeptical individual, so it was really very much a surprise to discover that this seems to be the case. The wines are the most procyanidin-rich I have encountered. The explanation seems to be the Tannat grape, which is grown widely here. The Madiran appellation requires at least 40 percent Tannat, but it is not uncommon to find wines that are 100 percent Tannat; the other grapes permitted in the blend are Cabernet Sauvignon, Cabernet Franc, and a local grape called Fer, or Pinenc. Tannat also features in other wines from southwest France: Côtes de Saint-Mont (at least 60 percent Tannat), Béarn, Irouléguy, and Tursan and, as a minor component, in Côtes du Brulhois. I have focused on Madiran and the red wines of Côtes de Saint-Mont, both because of their high procyanidin content and because a number of dynamic and quality-conscious producers are steadily raising the profiles of these appellations.

The reputation of these wines has yet to spread very far. Even in France, many people think that all Madiran has to offer is rustic charm, with harsh tannins that suit the regional food. How wrong they are! But there is no mistaking, these wines are best with food, whether it is a rare steak or a hearty vegetable soup.

The appellation of Madiran is not far from the Pyrenees, which can be seen on a clear day. Almost every year there is an Indian summer lasting well into October, and this is why the slow-ripening Tannat grape does so well in this area.

In the twelfth century Benedictine monks founded an abbey at Madiran, and the reputation of the wine was spread by pilgrims en route to Santiago de Compostela—although it is unclear precisely when Tannat became the main grape variety in Madiran. The region was devastated by phylloxera in the nineteenth century, and it was only through the efforts of enthusiasts that the local grape varieties were kept going.

The wines of Madiran generally have a combined fermentation and maceration time of three weeks or more, which ensures good extraction of polyphenols—including procyanidins. The Tannat grape is so rich in anthocyanins that the wines are usually a deep red-purple color, sometimes almost black. When young they are fruity (hints of raspberry and black currant). As they age, some develop a whiff of spices. These are strong, intense, complex wines that generally are well structured, with long-lasting tannins and good acidity. Despite the high tannins, it is unusual to find more than a slight deposit in these wines, even when they are five years old or more. These wines age gracefully into treasures you will enjoy yet still provide substantially more than average amounts of procyanidins!

Modern Madiran is an evolving and improving wine. In this respect Patrick Ducournau (whose wines are sold under the labels Domaine

Mouréou and La Chapelle Lenclos) has been a key influence, with his development of micro-oxygenation. This technique entails bubbling minute amounts of oxygen through young wines at different stages of the winemaking process to produce a well-balanced structure and reduce the ferocity of the tannins—it is now widely used not just in Madiran, but also in Bordeaux and in other countries besides France. Precisely what chemical reactions are triggered by micro-oxygenation are still under investigation by specialized laboratories. Based on comparisons of wines that have been made by traditional methods with those that have undergone micro-oxygenation, it does not appear to reduce procyanidin levels to any noticeable extent, even though the wines are a lot smoother.

In the United Kingdom, I can buy Madiran wines from a small number of producers. My favorites are Cuvée Charles de Batz (Charles de Batz is better known as the musketeer d'Artagnan) from Domaine Berthoumieu and Chapelle Lenclos from Domaine Mouréou. Both producers are members of Altema, an alliance of independent Madiran winemakers. When I visited the region in September 2005, I spent a pleasant afternoon at an Altema open day and tasting. I have not analyzed every wine I tasted—there are eighteen Altema members and some produce more than one cuvée—but I would expect them all to get ♥♥♥♥ or ♥♥♥♥♥ ratings for most vintages. There may be some exceptions for the 2003 vintage because the grapes ripened more quickly during the hot summer and the wines often show less acidity and smoother tannins than those from more typical vintages. Among those I particularly enjoyed and which rated highly in my analysis are: Château d'Aydie ♥♥♥♥♥, Domaine Dou Bernès ♥♥♥♥♥♥, Domaine Berthoumieu (Haute Tradition ♥♥♥♥ and Cuvée Charles de Batz ♥♥♥♥♥♥), Clos Basté ♥♥♥♥♥♥, Domaine Labranche Laffont ♥♥♥♥♥, Domaine Laougué ♥♥♥♥♥, Domaine Mouréou (Domaine Mouréou and Chapelle Lenclos ♥♥♥♥♥), and Château de Viella ♥♥♥♥♥.

Alain Brumont worked hard to raise the profile of Madiran during the 1980s and 1990s, and has a well-earned reputation for attention to detail, from vineyard to bottling. His best-known Madirans are bottled under the Château Montus and Château Bouscassé labels. The regular cuvée of Château Montus, made from 80 percent Tannat and 20 percent Cabernet Sauvignon rated ♥♥♥♥♥, and Château Bouscassé Vieilles Vignes (100 percent Tannat, unfined, unfiltered) rated ♥♥♥♥.

The quality-focused cooperative Producteurs Plaimont produces a range of Madiran, Côtes de Saint-Mont, and various Vins de Pays, both red and white. The cooperative's Directeur Général, André Dubosc, has united the members of this cooperative into an impressively well-organized group of producers determined to get the best from the region's grapes. The yield from vines used for Madiran and Côtes de Saint-Mont wines is restricted in order to give concentrated flavors. Harvesting by hand (a compulsory requirement for Côtes de Saint-Mont wines) means that only the best grapes are used. In the wineries modern technology such as micro-oxygenation is combined with key features of traditional methods—such as long maceration—to ensure outstanding wines with the authentic character of the region.

The following are some of the best Madirans I have found from Producteurs Plaimont. All achieve ♥♥♥♥ or ♥♥♥♥♥ ratings in most years, with procyanidin levels declining slightly six or seven years after the vintage. Château Vieila Village is a good wine for new converts, as it is somewhat lighter in style than many Madirans; it is made from 50 percent Tannat and 50 percent Cabernet Sauvignon. Plénitude (80 percent Tannat, 20 percent Cabernet Franc and/or Cabernet Sauvignon) is also very approachable. Château de Crouseilles and Château d'Arricau-Bordes (both 80 percent Tannat, 20 percent Cabernet Franc) are of very high quality.

Château de Sabazan, Château Saint-Go, Château du Bascou, and Le Faîte de Saint-Mont are all ♥♥♥♥ to ♥♥♥♥♥ Côtes de Saint-Mont wines from Producteurs Plaimont.

8

MODERATION
IS THE MESSAGE

THE HORRORS OF alcoholism and binge drinking invariably make bigger headlines than the good news about the health benefits of wine. While governments try to curb the worst drinking behaviors of their citizens, is it wise for any health professional to recommend daily wine consumption? I never advocate unrestrained intake. My recommendations are for moderate drinking of wines that have a high concentration of procyanidins—and I suggest that they accompany food. If this advice is followed, then drinking wine is likely to confer greater health benefit than not drinking it. But I have also analyzed a range of polyphenol-rich foods and alcohol-free drinks (see Chapter 4), so that nobody need feel they are obliged to drink wine every day.

GOOD DRINKING HABITS

The World Health Organization recently reported that when assessed in terms of its global burden of disease (death and disability), the harm from alcohol was coming close to that from tobacco. (Even though obesity causes more deaths than alcohol, as a burden of disease it ranks lower because less disability is attributed to obesity.) This raises concerns that all alcoholic beverages will be grouped together and labeled as the demon drink. The last thing any wine drinker wants is global restrictions on all alcoholic products; in that scenario, the antialcohol lobby would make no distinction between wine drinkers and consumers of alcopops (drinks such as alcoholic lemonade) and high-strength lagers.

From the research summarized in Chapter 2 it is clear that wine drinkers tend to have a diet and lifestyle that provide more health benefits than those of beer or spirits drinkers. As long as wine is seen to confer health benefits, it is less likely to be a target for public health officials. However, it is important that wine drinkers recognize the need to drink responsibly as part of a healthy lifestyle; traditionally this means that wine is mainly consumed with food.

Drinking wine with food generally has a moderating effect. A bottle is likely to be shared. If wine is chosen to complement a particular course, it may be inappropriate to continue drinking wine when that course is finished. But perhaps most importantly, food slows the absorption of alcohol, so levels of alcohol in the blood are lower than if the same amount is drunk on an empty stomach. In addition, if a meal is eaten slowly, wine consumption may be spread over an hour or more. This gives the body the chance to metabolize a fair proportion of the alcohol before the meal is finished. To keep alcohol consumption at a sensible level, go easy on the aperitifs and cut out the digestifs.

Many red wines today are made in a style that makes them easy to drink without food. But these wines do not confer the same health benefits as traditionally made, higher-tannin wines—and it makes no sense to quaff large quantities of wine in the belief that there is no risk to health.

However much one enjoys the conviviality of social drinking, it doesn't take much to exceed a safe intake of alcohol. A couple of drinks can soon lead to a reckless disregard for the notion of moderation. Know your limits! Depending on height, weight, sex, age, medical history, and ability to metabolize alcohol, an individual's safe limit of consumption may be very different from that of somebody else in their peer group. So it is very hard to generalize on what are safe limits. Public health bodies have made various recommendations—let's take a look at current guidelines.

WHAT IS safe DRINKING?

To understand the language of moderate consumption, it is important to know what is meant by "a drink" and "a unit of alcohol." Different countries have different ways of defining a safe intake of alcohol; in this definition safe means unlikely to cause harmful effects to health. But anybody who is planning to drive or operate any type of machinery should avoid alcohol completely.

In the United States, a standard unit contains 14 grams of pure alcohol: This is found in a 5-ounce glass of wine, a 12-ounce glass of beer, or a 1.5-ounce shot of spirits. The safe level for a man is defined as two drinks a day, and for a woman one drink a day. This represents a slightly lower alcohol intake for both men and women than the United Kingdom, but in practice it is very similar advice.

In the United Kingdom, alcohol consumption generally is assessed in units of alcohol. A unit of alcohol is defined as 8 grams of pure alcohol. Half a pint of beer with 3.5 percent ABV (Alcohol by Volume) represents one unit. A small (4-ounce) glass of wine with 12 percent ABV is 1.5 units. But these days we are far more likely to be offered a 6-ounce glass of wine that has 14 percent ABV—which as a single drink provides 2.5 units of alcohol. The U.K. government advises men not to exceed 3 to 4 units a day, and women not to exceed 2 to 3 units. This represents an upper limit of slightly less than three small glasses of wine a day (no more than half a bottle) for a man—and two small glasses for a woman. If you drink wine the French way—a small glass of wine of moderate (say, 12.5 percent) alcohol content with lunch, and the rest of your daily allowance with your evening meal—you should be within safe limits.

Recommendations for safe drinking are similar in many countries. In France and Denmark, large population studies have generally shown no harmful effects at this level of daily wine drinking, or even with slightly higher consumption. But in France, Italy, and other wine-producing countries in southern Europe, wine is mainly drunk with food, at both lunch and dinner. So levels of alcohol in the bloodstream of consumers who keep to guidelines for moderate drinking rarely will reach harmful levels. It is important to bear this in mind when reading reports of the relationship between wine consumption in these places and deaths from heart disease or other causes. The overall daily amount consumed without causing harm may appear high, but this does not imply that it is safe to drink such amounts on an empty stomach during one short after-work binge.

It occasionally has been said to me in jest: "I've been following your advice and drinking two glasses of wine a day, but I find that I now wake up each morning with a terrible hangover!" Of course the joke is that these individuals are adding two glasses of wine on top of whatever else they may be drinking routinely. To avoid any element of doubt, it is total daily alcohol consumption that is important. So if you decide to become a wine drinker you need to curtail your other drinking habits.

Alcohol can adversely affect sports performance and may be dangerous, for example when swimming, diving, or skiing. This is something people often forget in vacation situations, sometimes with tragic consequences.

Irrespective of whether wine consumption confers health benefits, some people should not drink any alcohol:

- Women in the first trimester (twelve weeks) of pregnancy, those who think they might be pregnant, or are not taking precautions and could become pregnant. U.K. guidelines advise that in the last two trimesters pregnant women should limit their alcohol intake to no more than one 4-ounce glass of wine with food, once or twice a week.
- Anyone taking prescription or over-the-counter medication that might interact with alcohol.
- Anyone who has difficulty restricting their intake to moderate levels or has a history of excess alcohol consumption.

PROTECTING YOUR HEART WITH A REGULAR GLASS OF WINE

Excessive alcohol consumption can damage heart muscle, and this eventually may lead to heart failure. On the other hand, the most common cause of heart failure is myocardial infarction (heart attack) as a result of coronary heart disease—and regular moderate alcohol consumption decreases the number of heart attacks. This raises the question of whether regular moderate drinking is more likely to cause heart failure or prevent it.

The Framingham Heart Study is one of the most important studies of risk factors for coronary heart disease. The study started in 1948 and involved 5,209 residents of Framingham, Massachusetts. In 1971 the offspring of the original participants and their spouses were also included in the survey. The effect of alcohol consumption on the occurrence of congestive heart failure was determined from information collected up to 1995. Compared to nondrinkers, heart failure was less common in men at all levels of moderate alcohol consumption. The same protection was not seen in women. However, neither men nor women showed an increased level of heart failure at any level of alcohol consumption. But excessive drinking among the Framingham participants was rare, so it was difficult to assess what level of excessive drinking is likely to lead to heart failure. Other studies have shown that damage to the heart muscle generally occurs with five or more drinks a day.

Moderate consumption of alcohol reduces the overall risk of heart disease. From studies of wine drinkers the greatest benefit is seen for people drinking one or two small glasses a day. Many people seem to assume that they can drink moderately for four days of the week and then increase their consumption on the weekends and still benefit. However, a number of studies have reported that binge drinking cancels out the benefits of moderate consumption.

Bouts of excess drinking on vacation, or at parties and other celebrations can also cause an abnormal heart beat (arrhythmia), which can be sudden in onset and life threatening. Although fairly uncommon, individual sensitivity to this effect is variable, and in some people it may occur at levels of drinking that are just slightly above moderate levels. If it occurs once, it is likely to happen again, so you need to reduce substantially the amount you drink or abstain in the future.

For some studies that have reported the harmful consequences of excessive drinking, it seems likely that other diet and lifestyle factors have also contributed. For instance, the CARDIA Study conducted in California followed young adults to define risk factors that contribute to coronary heart disease. Coronary atherosclerosis was assessed after fifteen years, when the participants were aged thirty-three to forty-five. Binge drinkers had significantly more evidence of heart disease. No breakdown was provided for red wine drinkers in comparison to nondrinkers or other drinkers. In general, the more alcohol consumed the more likely it was to find evidence of silent (asymptomatic) heart disease. However, almost 70 percent of the participants were either overweight or obese, so other dietary and lifestyle factors probably contributed to the occurrence of premature heart disease.

In many respects this Californian study highlights the difficulties of comparing one country or region to another. While many young Europeans in France, Spain, and Italy, for example, may be brought up drinking red wine, in other countries wine generally is not the first choice of alcoholic drink. If, as our research shows, the procyanidins in red wine have important protective properties, moderate consumption of wine is likely to confer benefit in terms of improved blood vessel function from an early age. The consequence of this would be to delay initial changes within blood vessels that precede atherosclerotic lesion formation. So if a similar study to the Californian CARDIA study was undertaken in southwest France, different results might be obtained.

wine as a LIFeSTYLe CHOICe

In the United Kingdom, Australia, and certain other countries, units of alcohol or other health guidelines may be printed on wine labels, but currently there is no legal requirement for wine producers or retailers to include this information.

In the United States, legislation passed in 1988 required labels to warn consumers of the adverse effects of alcohol. In 1995, the U.S. wine industry requested permission to allow labels to carry a statement that moderate consumption of alcoholic beverages may reduce the risk of heart disease. In 2003, after a lengthy consultation process, it was agreed that certain directional guidance would be permitted. The final decision to exclude specific claims of health benefit from wine labeling was the only possible course for the government, given the lack of detailed testing of specific wines through clinical trials, and in view of the fact that a moderate amount of wine for one individual may be excessive for another. Permissible directional guidance includes referring the consumer to their family doctor for advice and referring them to Federal Dietary Guidelines.

Unfortunately, the Dietary Guidelines for Americans 2005 (DGA2005) are not exactly an insightful read when it comes to wine. There is some acceptance that moderate alcohol consumption may benefit some middle-aged and elderly people. That is a very conservative view, particularly if procyanidin-rich red wines can play an important part in preserving the healthy function of blood vessels throughout life. But the general tone of

DGA2005 toward alcohol consumption can be inferred from the statement that "Abstention is an important option." Apparently 45 percent of adult Americans do not drink any alcohol.

Obesity and diabetes is an ever-increasing problem in many countries. In the United States, for example, it is estimated that 65 percent of Americans are overweight, 30 percent are obese, and 7 percent have diabetes. The Guidelines consider all alcohol consumption as a source of excess calories—much like sugar and saturated fat. Yet wine drinkers tend to be leaner than non-wine drinkers and are generally healthier; and it is important to note that they are less likely to suffer from type 2 diabetes. So perhaps a better informed comment on wine as part of a lifestyle pattern of moderate drinking with food would be more helpful.

Corporate America also has a problem with wine. It is obsessed by the idea that somebody might sue because they consumed a complementary glass of wine and then suffered an untoward event, which would not have occurred if they hadn't accepted that wine. I have attended receptions where the only way

TAKING A DAY OFF

I am often asked whether it is a good idea to avoid alcohol completely for two or three days a week. I very much doubt whether this happens in the long-living populations who drink procyanidin-rich wine with their food. Research shows that moderate wine drinkers (two to three small glasses of wine a day) have the lowest mortality from all causes with no increased risk of cirrhosis of the liver. Many of the beneficial effects of alcohol (raising HDL-cholesterol levels, reducing risk of blood clots, actions on endothelial function) are transient; therefore, it makes sense to follow a pattern of moderate daily drinking. However, if on a daily basis you exceed safe levels of drinking, then this is more likely to lead to cirrhosis. Having two or three days off between these drunken excesses will allow your liver to recover to some extent, but a better choice is to drink only in moderation. Then daily drinking no longer will be so damaging to your health. Also be aware that drinkers who smoke have more than double the risk of cirrhosis compared to nonsmokers.

to have a glass of wine is to shuffle into a dark corner of the room and pay for the privilege. Yet at the same time, tables are piled high with cheese, crackers, dips, and other snacks, and you can drink as many bottles of sugary soft drinks as you like. I think this is part of the obesity problem! A glass of wine with some nuts and olives would be a healthier choice.

HEALTH RISKS FROM EXCESS ALCOHOL

Everybody should be aware of the problems of excess alcohol consumption. Cirrhosis of the liver is untreatable and eventually fatal. The number of people dying from liver cirrhosis is steadily rising around the world. This is a warning that too many people, particularly in younger age groups, are drinking in excess.

Alcohol consumption is rising more rapidly in young women than men, both in the United States and Europe. Datamonitor, a London-based market research company, has reported that at the current rate of increase, by the year 2009, eighteen- to twenty-four-year-old women will be drinking three large (8.5-ounce) glasses of wine (or equivalent)—9 to 10 units of alcohol—a day. Because this level of drinking frequently occurs among women who do not eat healthily, this group is at very high risk of alcoholic liver damage. The threat of breast cancer is also much increased by this level of drinking. Many of the harmful effects of excess alcohol can be reversed by a prolonged period of abstinence, although it is not yet known whether the risk of breast cancer returns to the level of nondrinkers. But cirrhosis is a real danger because it is irreversible.

Wine drinkers have been reported to have less cirrhosis than consumers of beer or spirits drinking a similar amount of alcohol. This survey was based on 30,630 Danes, including 14,335 women. I think this is likely to reflect a completely different pattern of drinking. Wine drinkers who experience the greatest benefit for the most part consume their daily quota with meals. This slows the rate at which alcohol enters the bloodstream and leads to lower concentrations in the blood. This is likely to be a key protective mechanism, since it means the liver and other tissues are less likely to be exposed to harmful concentrations of alcohol. In addition, the procyanidins in red wine may exert a protective effect on liver cells, so that the liver is more resistant to the injurious effects of the absorbed alcohol. For some it will be interesting to know that drinking coffee (four cups a day) has been linked to lower levels of cirrhosis in both drinkers and nondrinkers, indicating that coffee may have some protective properties.

One of the reasons the liver is more at risk than other tissues is that when alcohol is absorbed from the stomach and duodenum, it passes directly to the liver via the hepatic portal vein. This can result in higher alcohol concentrations in this blood vessel, which therefore hit the liver harder before it passes into the rest of the circulating blood and becomes diluted.

As part of a routine medical examination, your doctor may decide to measure your liver function. This is done via a blood test to measure levels of liver enzymes in your blood; if higher than normal in someone who drinks alcohol on a regular basis, this indicates that they are exceeding a safe level of drinking and causing damage to their liver. However, even among moderate to heavy drinkers individual sensitivity to these blood tests may vary. For anyone who is balancing their nighttime excesses against the severity of their morning hangover, a word of warning—you are exceeding safe limits and may be risking your life!

Excess alcohol consumption also causes brain damage, and women are at greater risk than men. Other harmful effects of excess alcohol, such as heart failure, muscle degeneration, and liver disease also occur at a lower level of alcohol consumption in women than in men. That is why the limits for safe drinking are set lower for women than men.

KEEPING AN EYE ON BLOOD PRESSURE

Although moderate alcohol consumption is widely seen as a protective factor for coronary heart disease, if consumption is above the moderate level of two drinks a day, it can cause high blood pressure, which in turn increases the risk of heart disease. It is a fine line to tread! Some individuals are more sensitive than others to this side effect of their daily tipple. If you are overweight or do not exercise, these habits can lead to higher blood pressure, so excess drinking will only make this worse.

Several studies have looked at drinking habits and the risk of high blood pressure. A detailed study in 2004 showed that drinking mainly with meals was less likely to cause high blood pressure than drinking without food. In addition, wine drinkers were less likely to suffer high blood pressure than beer or liquor (spirits) drinkers. An Italian study also looked at the impact of drinking patterns on blood pressure. This study was extended to assess long-term effects on health. It found that high blood pressure was more frequent, even for wine drinkers, if wine was not consumed with meals. Over the long term, the habit of drinking other than with meals was linked to a higher number of deaths from all causes. In other words, any protective effects from regular wine drinking are lost if it is not combined with food.

DRINKING TO a HeaLTHY FUTURe!

Some studies have come to the conclusion that moderate alcohol consumption provides little, if any, health benefit for younger people. I cannot see how this can be true in terms of the beneficial effects of procyanidin-rich red wines. If high procyanidin intake ensures healthy blood vessels that are resistant to atherosclerosis, then it is important that modest consumption is sustained throughout adult life, even if the benefits are not apparent until middle or old age. Conversely, if you drink only water or soft drinks until you retire, there is no evidence that you can become a wine drinker and gain the same protection against heart disease or dementia in old age.

Health claims are considered misleading if they cannot be backed up with scientific or medical evidence. My original objectives when I started research on red wine were to discover which components of wine were most important for protecting and improving blood vessel function, and whether all wines conferred the same health benefit. Our research indicates the key role of dietary procyanidins in modifying blood vessel function. We have also discovered that wines from areas where people are living longer contain much higher levels of procyanidins than typical wines from other areas. The association of particular types of wine with areas of increased longevity suggests that procyanidins make an important contribution to long-term vascular well-being.

A general principle of treating any disease is that the dose of medicine should be sufficient to control symptoms without causing any harmful side effects. In the case of procyanidins, if the ideal dose can be achieved with a smaller amount of wine, then less alcohol will be consumed. Hence the advantage for health from procyanidin-rich wines is clear. There is concern among health authorities in some countries that the link between reduced heart disease and regular wine drinking "should not encourage people to drink or to increase alcohol consumption for health reasons." I would like to think that my recommendations for drinking procyanidin-rich wines might actually help some people reduce their alcohol consumption.

9

seven diet myths that put your health at risk

You often hear people saying they wouldn't want to grow old if they were to suffer from such and such an illness—meaning any disease that diminishes their faculties, reduces their independence, or affects their quality of life. We are becoming increasingly aware that what we eat and the lifestyle we lead affect our long-term health: We can make a positive effort to avoid ill health in the future by adopting good habits from an early age.

Healthy eating throughout your life is the best route to living longer. This is because diet and chronic diseases such as heart disease and cancer are closely linked. Obesity is one of the most serious health issues facing the world today: It is linked to type 2 diabetes, various forms of cancer, high blood pressure, and coronary heart disease, and it exacerbates the problems associated with arthritis. Typical problems of old age such as blindness, osteoporosis, cognitive decline, and dementia are also affected by diet and general physical condition. Avoiding these disabling diseases will maximize quality of life and allow older people to maintain their independence.

Although avoiding obesity is important, losing weight is not the only consideration for long-term good health. The underlying drive for changing what you eat should be: "What do I need to do to have a healthier and longer life?" Fad diets, which promise weight loss by restricting the type of food you eat, are not the answer. A healthy nutrition plan means eating a variety of natural, tasty, satisfying foods. Gradual weight change is best, as it is more likely to achieve a lasting result. It may take one to two years of progressive weight loss to achieve your ideal weight. The goal should be a diet that improves health first and foremost, and weight loss will then follow over time. This is the strategy I am recommending to you.

In this chapter I examine some diet myths and fads that might be putting your health at risk: I want to heighten awareness of dietary factors that increase the risk of illness. A lifestyle aimed at long-term well-being is vital for everyone, irrespective of their weight. There is no room for complacency.

MYTH 1: SUGAR CONSUMPTION DOES NOT CAUSE OBESITY OR DIABETES

Less a diet myth, more a blatant lie from the food industry, which claims that there is insufficient evidence linking sugar consumption with obesity, diabetes, and other health problems—and that sugar is added to products simply to satisfy consumer tastes. Well, for the record, I consider current levels of sugar consumption to be one of the biggest, if not the biggest, health risk to people of all ages. This is particularly true for children, who do not recognize the dangers. In terms of calorie-rich, nutrient-poor food, refined sugar is the chief culprit: It provides calories and nothing else—not a trace of vitamins or minerals. In a society that consumes more energy than it expends, reducing sugar consumption has to be a primary goal.

The pro-sugar lobby is immensely powerful. It has attempted to discredit any report that recommends reduced sugar intake or the introduction of legislation to limit the amount of sugar added to food. Its power is such that governments frequently have been diverted from these issues. For many years even the World Health Organization (WHO) came out less strongly on the sugar issue than might have been expected. This seems to have been due to underhand influences, since it has been widely reported that food industry lobbyists managed to infiltrate WHO committees with scientists sympathetic to their opinions. WHO, with the Food and Agriculture Organization (FAO) of the United Nations, started to set matters straight in 2003 with a report by a committee of experts on "Diet, Nutrition and the Prevention of Chronic Diseases." In 2004 WHO put forward its "Global Strategy on Diet, Physical Activity and Health," which included recommendations that advertisements aimed at children for sugar-rich foods and beverages be banned. It also encouraged governments to introduce fiscal policies that would influence food choices.

A sugar tax seems an excellent idea, as I find it quite remarkable that most people seem willing to ignore the problems sugar consumption is causing. If the price of every sweet dessert and sugared drink was increased for every gram of added sugar, consumers would think twice before buying. If governments are reluctant to tax sugar, they could at least insist on labeling that includes health warnings of the risks of excess sugar consumption.

If you are even slightly overweight, you should think about whether you might be at risk of diabetes. Many people who develop diabetes because of their diet and lack of exercise are in a prediabetic state—so-called syndrome X—for many years, but their bodies just about keep the symptoms hidden. Common symptoms in people who are on the point of becoming diabetic, whatever the cause, are excessive thirst and a more frequent need to urinate.

Diabetes mellitus, to give the disease its correct name, has two forms: type 1 diabetes, which is also sometimes called juvenile onset or insulin-dependent diabetes; and type 2 diabetes, which has also been called non-insulin-dependent diabetes mellitus (sometimes abbreviated to NIDDM) or maturity onset diabetes.

Type 1 diabetes is the less common form. The symptoms often first appear in susceptible individuals when they are children or teenagers, but they may occur later in life. It is not related to being overweight. Frequently it has been linked to viral infections, which lead to the immune system destroying the cells in the pancreas that produce insulin. Insulin is the hormone that controls sugar levels in the blood by stimulating tissues such as muscle and fat to transport sugar into cells and so remove it from the circulating blood. Clearly, if the pancreas no longer produces insulin, then insulin will need to be administered—hence the term insulin-dependent diabetes. This type of diabetes is likely to have a very sudden onset, sometimes with life-threatening symptoms. Blood sugar can be controlled with two or more injections of insulin per day.

Type 2 diabetes was once known as maturity onset diabetes because it occurred mainly in middle-aged and elderly people. This is no longer an appropriate term, because more and more young adults and teenagers are developing this disease. Nor is non-insulin-dependent diabetes an accurate description. It is true that initially it often can be controlled with oral medicines, but depending on the duration or severity of the disease, the pancreas may fail and stop producing sufficient insulin. Then it becomes necessary to inject insulin to control blood sugar levels in the same way as for type 1 diabetes.

If you are overweight, you are at risk of developing type 2 diabetes: 80 to 90 percent of patients with this form of diabetes are overweight or obese. It is a mistake to think of type 2 diabetes as a mild form of illness. It is linked to just as many, if not more, long-term health problems and complications as type 1 diabetes.

If diabetes is suspected, your doctor will measure your blood sugar levels after an overnight fast to discover whether they are higher than normal. However, this may not be conclusive, because your fasting blood sugar levels may be close to normal. Before diabetes occurs there may be many years when you are in a prediabetic state, where your body struggles to control blood sugar levels after a meal. This may be because your pancreas has been working too hard and is now failing to produce sufficient insulin, or you may be suffering from insulin resistance (also known as syndrome X or metabolic syndrome). This is when the cells in muscle, fat, and the liver that normally would respond to insulin by rapidly taking sugar out of the circulating blood lose their insulin sensitivity and fail to respond. Blood sugar levels then remain high for several hours after a meal before slowly coming down to healthy levels.

The sugar that circulates in the blood is glucose. A glucose tolerance test can assess insulin resistance as a symptom of a prediabetic state. After an overnight fast a drink containing 75 grams (2.5 ounces) of glucose is consumed and blood glucose levels are measured two hours later to see if they are within the healthy range. A person with higher than normal healthy levels is said to have impaired glucose tolerance.

Two and a half ounces of glucose is quite a lot—it's the equivalent of fifteen teaspoons of sugar. A typical soft drink that is sweetened with sugar contains seven to eight teaspoons in a 12-ounce serving, so it is not surprising that regular consumption of soft drinks is so often linked to diabetes and obesity, particularly in children. Drinking several sweet drinks a day puts a tremendous strain on the pancreas because of the repeated high demands for insulin to cope with the sugar load. Eventually, the pancreas cannot meet the demands placed on it, and diabetes sets in. This is hastened by cells becoming less responsive to insulin. Several studies have concluded that excess consumption of sugar-sweetened beverages is a major factor in type 2 diabetes in young people. Cutting out foods and drinks with added sugar should be a priority for everybody.

If you already have cut out sweet foods and drinks, then an exercise program is essential to help reduce insulin resistance. Exercise encourages cells to take up sugar from the bloodstream and lowers the need for insulin.

An elevated amount of sugar in the circulating blood is a key factor leading to blood vessel damage during the prediabetic state and in patients with poorly controlled diabetes, which in turn triggers a whole range of vascular complications in later years. Persistently elevated blood glucose levels cause damage to protein molecules in your blood and inside your body's cells. The damaged proteins (sometimes called advanced glycation end products or AGEs) have toxic effects on arteries throughout the body, increasing not only the risk of heart disease from deposits of oxidized LDL-cholesterol, but also the likelihood of Alzheimer's disease. Other studies have shown that the body may recognize AGEs as foreign bodies, triggering inflammatory responses.

High sugar levels also affect the endothelium (the inner lining of cells that protect each blood vessel). This can reduce vasodilation (normal, healthy relaxation and widening of blood vessels) and increase the likelihood of high blood pressure and the formation of blood clots. A person diagnosed with type 2 diabetes may have had abnormally high blood sugar levels for many years before diagnosis, so perhaps it is not surprising that type 2 diabetes is often associated with coronary heart disease. In fact, diabetes often remains undiagnosed until after a heart attack.

The factors that increase the development of coronary atherosclerosis affect other arteries in the body, and diabetes is also linked to a higher occurrence of stroke and peripheral vascular disease. Uncontrolled diabetes can also result in impotence, kidney problems, nerve damage, and blindness. What is the solution? Quite frankly, these problems are very difficult to treat. Radical changes in diet and lifestyle before they occur are the best long-term option—the sooner the better.

Obesity is also associated with an increased risk of some cancers, including cancer of the breast, prostate, colon, and rectum. It seems unlikely that this is simply a direct effect of obesity but more likely the result of various dietary and lifestyle factors. Smoking is the most common cause of cancer, but dietary factors are the second most common cause, perhaps contributing to as much as 30 percent of all cancers. Excess consumption of sugar or certain other foods might be the link. Certainly, eating calorie-rich meals that lack important micronutrients seems likely to contribute to the risk of cancer, because the cellular mechanisms that normally resist cancerous changes may no longer work sufficiently well.

MYTH 2: FOLLOWING A LOW-FAT DIET IS THE BEST WAY TO LOSE WEIGHT AND STAY HEALTHY

This myth has been spread by government bodies, nutritionists, and the food industry for almost thirty years. A generation of consumers has grown up obsessed with reducing the fat content of their food, yet with no understanding of the importance of different types of fat in the diet, and with a belief that carbohydrates are somehow better than fats.

In the 1970s there was thought to be sufficient evidence linking consumption of saturated fat to heart disease that governments started to recommend the restriction of fat intake. It was considered too complex a health message to point out that only saturated fat might be harmful—or to explain that a combination of saturated and unsaturated fats is found in all kinds of food, whether butter, olive oil, cheese, or meat. Indications that diets based mainly on monounsaturated and polyunsaturated were healthy ones were ignored. The "health" advice was to restrict all fat consumption. So fatty foods like nuts and avocados were labeled as unhealthful; some health organizations still have not updated this advice and still recommend that people should avoid these foods, particularly if they want to lose weight. All fat contains twice as many calories per gram as carbohydrate and protein, but the argument that nuts and avocados are high in calories ignores the evidence that the fats they contain are healthy fats, and they also contribute valuable vitamins and minerals as part of a healthful pattern of eating.

For better health everybody was advised to restrict fat consumption and eat more foods rich in carbohydrate. This has to be seen as the biggest health blunder of the twentieth century and yet many authorities are still unwilling to admit they were wrong. What is worse is that the food industry has created a juggernaut of low-fat and reduced-fat foods that are very high in sugar and other processed carbohydrates. When low-fat diets were first advocated there was no evidence that people living on such diets for long periods of time had lower levels of heart disease, let alone obesity and diabetes. I think it is time to end this experiment and accept that these diets have not resulted in improved health and long-term well-being.

Why have low-fat high-carbohydrate diets failed? There seems to be a number of reasons why diets based on reducing fat intake and eating more carbohydrate-based foods have not worked in the long term. If the advice about carbohydrates had been more specific, and had focused on whole-grain and natural foods, the problem may not have been so severe, but thirty years ago the study of the glycemic index (GI) and glycemic load (GL) was in its infancy. Glycemic index literally means the sugar index, and refers to the readily absorbable sugars present in a food. The higher the rate of absorption of sugars into the blood, the higher the glycemic index. Refined starchy foods such as white bread, and some readily digestible starches like white rice and potatoes, have almost the same glycemic index as pure sugar. Glycemic load refers to the total digestible sugar in a given portion of food. The higher the GI and GL the greater the amount of sugars a meal provides. Rapid absorption of sugars causes insulin production to rise rapidly. This stimulates tissues to take the sugar out of the blood. But this can occur so rapidly that sugar levels may dip. This leads to the sensation of still being hungry. So refined carbohydrates (starches and sugars) do not satisfy the appetite; rather, they tend to stimulate compulsive eating.

The failure of low-fat diets has caused the diet industry to switch its emphasis from low fat to low GI. Low-GI foods are those that contain either no or few carbohydrates—such as fish, shellfish, poultry, meat, eggs, cheese, and most vegetables—or that contain slowly absorbed carbohydrates, such as nuts, beans, pulses, and unrefined whole-grain products. This is a positive step, but it is important to remember that low GI is not the same as low carb. Carbohydrates have a place in a healthy diet, and finding the right balance of carbohydrates from slowly absorbed foods should be the goal.

Because of the recent interest in low-carb and low-GI diets, a number of studies have investigated how refined carbohydrates affect eating habits. Researchers have found that obese subjects tend to eat fewer calories when their carbohydrate intake is restricted. A reduction in carbohydrate may make losing weight easier than a reduction in fat or protein. It is not only the glycemic index but the total amount of carbohydrate—the glycemic load—that needs careful management.

Excess saturated fat consumption is linked to an increased level of heart disease. The explanation put forward, and still widely accepted, is that eating too much saturated fat leads to high levels of potentially harmful LDL-cholesterol in the blood. This is often considered to be the single most important trigger for heart disease. It is hard to refute the role of LDL-cholesterol in the processes of atherosclerosis—except that in many of the largest health surveys where high levels of LDL-cholesterol have been recorded in subjects with heart disease, there is often a similar number of people without heart disease who have roughly equivalent levels of LDL-cholesterol. Heart disease also occurs in many people with low or healthy levels of LDL-cholesterol. So it is not such a straightforward relationship. This suggests that some people are protected through their genes or other factors from the adverse consequences of raised LDL-cholesterol.

At the same time that we were told to stop eating fat, we were advised that foods that are high in cholesterol, such as eggs, shellfish, and liver, should be avoided in order to help reduce blood cholesterol levels. Research has since shown that cholesterol in food is poorly absorbed in the intestines, so the effects of cholesterol-rich foods are less significant than originally thought. In fact, the body is very good at making all the cholesterol it needs. Cell membranes, the fatty layers that hold a cell together, are rich in cholesterol, so each cell has its own cholesterol management system to maintain cholesterol at optimal levels. If the foods you eat do not contain what your body assesses to be the right amount of fat or cholesterol, your liver will produce them from carbohydrate.

One of the reasons why low-fat diets originally were encouraged was that it was found that blood cholesterol levels were lower on such diets. Further

CAN HEALTHY FAT CONSUMPTION HELP YOU LOSE BODY FAT?

The high-profile Atkins diet has stimulated a lot of research into the mechanisms of weight loss and the effects of different types of diet. Some fascinating insights have been published.

One study looked at the effect of low-calorie low-carbohydrate diets on obese subjects with type 2 diabetes. This was compared with a low-calorie high-carbohydrate diet. Both diets provided approximately the same amount of calories from protein (25 to 26 percent of daily calories). The low-carbohydrate diet provided 39 percent of daily calories from carbohydrate and 35 percent from fat. So this was not an Atkins-style high-protein diet; it was more of a high-fat diet. For the high-carbohydrate diet the corresponding amounts were 62 percent from carbohydrate and 10 percent from fat. The ratio of saturated, monounsaturated, and polyunsaturated fatty acids were in roughly equal proportions in each diet.

After four weeks, subjects on both diets had similar decreases in body weight. However, insulin levels were down by 30 percent on the low-carbohydrate diet, indicating a reduction in insulin resistance. HDL-cholesterol ("good" cholesterol) increased by 15 percent on the low-carbohydrate diet but did not change on the high-carbohydrate diet. Visceral fat was reduced by more than 30 percent on the low-carbohydrate diet, and unchanged with the high-carbohydrate diet. This is an important observation because visceral fat—the fat in your abdomen around your intestines—is closely associated with the onset of insulin resistance and diabetes.

It is too early to conclude that excess carbohydrate is the cause of increased visceral fat, but the results of this study raise some interesting questions, particularly about the role fat consumption plays in fat accumulation in different parts of the body. Restricting carbohydrate intake while introducing a healthy level of fat consumption is likely to help correct metabolic abnormalities in some patients with obesity and diabetes. This forms part of my diet recommendations.

studies have shown that a large percentage of individuals following a low-fat, high-carbohydrate diet have only small decreases in their LDL-cholesterol levels, and a much greater reduction in HDL-cholesterol (the good, protective form of cholesterol). This means that such diets are potentially harmful—the risk of heart disease would be expected to increase rather than decrease on such a diet.

"Eating fat makes you fat" is a fallacy. Obesity is often equated with excess consumption of fat. This is a misconception. It is true that fatty foods have a higher calorie count than low-fat foods, but any excess energy (calorie/kilojoule) intake from carbohydrates is converted into fat in the body.

What is worse is that the main type of fat produced by the body from excess carbohydrates is a potentially harmful saturated fat, known as palmitic acid, which can adversely influence cholesterol levels. Worse still, for many individuals there is also an increase in pro-atherosclerotic lipid particles in the blood and increased triglycerides, as well as reduced HDL (good) cholesterol. So a low-fat high-carbohydrate diet can have an adverse effect on blood lipid profile, increasing the risk of heart disease.

Studies have shown that blood cholesterol and triglycerides can be improved by replacing saturated fat with mono- and polyunsaturated fats rather than with carbohydrate. Triglyceride levels are then lower, HDL-cholesterol higher, and LDL-cholesterol remains at about the same level. No more than 50 percent of energy intake from carbohydrates is probably optimal. Diets with a balance of fats are therefore best for long-term well-being. Replacing saturated fats with monounsaturated and polyunsaturated fats needs to be carefully managed. The majority of our fat intake should ideally be from monounsaturated fats, but in industrialized countries a predominance of foods high in omega-6 polyunsaturated fatty acids (PUFAs) with low omega-3 PUFAs has been linked to oxidation and free radical formation, resulting in increased atherosclerosis.

Consuming too much carbohydrate can also affect the ability of heart and skeletal muscle to use fatty acids as a source of energy. The body uses fats to provide 60 to 80 percent of the energy needed by our muscles, particularly during exercise and periods of fasting. Meals and snacks rich in carbohydrate have the effect of suppressing the use of fats for energy production. So to burn fat between meals it is important to avoid snacking on large amounts of carbohydrate. You will gain the most benefit in terms of improving your blood triglycerides if you avoid sugary snacks and sweetened drinks before you exercise.

The ill-informed advice to restrict all fat consumption was compounded by recommendations to replace butter (which contains 54 percent saturated fat) with margarine and reduced-fat spreads, because they are made from vegetable fats and contain a lower proportion of saturated fat. The first piece of advice has been a disaster; the second turned it into a health care catastrophe of even greater significance.

To create a butter substitute, vegetable oil needs to be solid or semisolid. To achieve this, vegetable oils are hydrogenated, which entails bubbling hydrogen gas through the oils in the presence of toxic chemical catalysts. Hydrogenated fat is largely composed of trans fats. This term refers to the modified chemical structure of the fat: In the process of hydrogenation the fat molecules are bent into the opposite direction to what naturally occurs; hence the term *trans fats*. Various other chemical processes are necessary to clean up these modified fats before they can be made into margarine. Coloring, flavoring, and preservatives to prevent it from oxidizing and becoming rancid are also added.

Are these products healthier than butter? Certainly not! The body finds it difficult to metabolize trans fat molecules. They accumulate in the bloodstream and increase the risk of atherosclerosis. When these fats get incorporated into cell membranes, the cells may no longer function normally, and consumption of trans fats has been linked to an increased risk of diabetes and cancer. By the early 1990s it was clear that hydrogenated fats, the dietary source of trans fats, were a major cause of increased heart disease in people who had switched to them for their health benefit. A high intake of hydrogenated fats is also associated with an increased risk of an irregular heartbeat (cardiac arrhythmia), which sometimes can be life threatening. It seems likely that hydrogenated fat is a more important cause of heart disease in our society than the consumption of saturated fat.

This is a prime example of why it is best to stick to natural products and avoid overmanipulated man-made "foods." Hydrogenated fats are still widely used in the food industry, in cakes, biscuits, crackers, and pastries, as well as in ready-made meals and other convenience foods. Fast food fries or chips are often cooked with hydrogenated fat. Several countries have already banned them; others will do so soon. My advice is never to buy foods containing hydrogenated fat.

Common sense is finally entering the arena of low-fat foods, but there is a long way to go to change the vested interests of the food industry, let alone consumers' habits. Thirty years of misinformation cannot be erased overnight.

CHOCOLATE AND CHOLESTEROL

Not all fats are equal when it comes to cholesterol synthesis in the body. The saturated fats with the greatest effects on increasing cholesterol levels are myristic and palmitic acid; these are high in meat and dairy products. Stearic acid, another saturated fat, does not adversely influence cholesterol levels. Chocolate is often given as an example of a fatty food that is bad for your health. It is certainly true that milk chocolate and other highly sweetened chocolate-flavored snack bars are not healthy choices. But dark chocolate is a different story. In fact, a typical analysis of cocoa fat reveals approximately 33 percent stearic acid (a healthy saturated fat), 35 percent oleic acid (a healthy monounsaturated fat), 27 percent palmitic acid (a potentially unhealthy saturated fat), 2 percent arachidic acid (a minor saturated fat), and 3 percent polyunsaturated fatty acid. So just over a quarter of the fat is likely to affect cholesterol adversely and the other fats are likely to counter this through neutral or beneficial actions.

Saturated fat is really not such a big issue with dark chocolate. Remember, however, that even moderate amounts of procyanidin-rich dark chocolate contribute calories to your overall daily intake. A serving of 1.75 ounces of chocolate provides at least 250 calories, more than 50 percent of which come from fat. Most types of dark chocolate also contain a substantial amount of sugar—usually about 10 to 15 grams in 1.75 ounces of chocolate.

MYTH 3: ATKINS-STYLE LOW-CARB HIGH-PROTEIN DIETS ARE BEST

Many people have successfully lost weight by following an Atkins-style diet, which focuses on protein and fat and avoids carbohydrate. Often the biggest weight loss is in the first six months. In comparative studies with other diets, the weight lost over one year is very similar. Dropout rates for all diets studied are high. Nevertheless low-carb diets have some passionate advocates. Unfortunately, the emphasis on eating meat, with a high intake of saturated fats, and restricted consumption of fruits and vegetables, puts you at risk of heart disease, cancer, gout (see page 143), and atherosclerosis. This is not an ideal strategy for sustained good health.

High consumption of animal protein (from meat and fish) puts you at risk of raised blood homocysteine levels. This can increase the risk of a number of problems, including heart disease, memory loss, and even Alzheimer's disease. Homocysteine is a metabolic breakdown product of methionine, an

WHAT IS GOUT? CAN I AVOID IT?

Gout is one of the most painful forms of arthritis. It is caused by the buildup of uric acid crystals in joints. The big toe is often affected first, but other joints commonly affected include the ankle, knee, foot, elbow, wrist, and hand. Obesity, insulin resistance, diabetes, high blood pressure, and kidney disease are all risk factors for gout. It is becoming more widespread, and this is thought to be explained by dietary and lifestyle trends.

High levels of uric acid in the blood are an indication that a person may be at risk of developing gout. Moderately raised uric acid levels are also linked with an increased risk of stroke and heart attack. So what is uric acid and where does it come from? It is a metabolic product from the breakdown of purines. Purines are compounds found in high levels in some foods; they are also generated as part of normal metabolism. They play a variety of roles in the body and are a component of the genetic information in every cell. Normally the kidneys are able to excrete excess uric acid, but in some people this does not occur efficiently, which leads to uric acid accumulation.

Dietary recommendations to avoid gout generally dictate avoiding purine-rich foods and alcohol. Findings from the Health Professionals Follow-up Study indicate the main risk factors for gout are eating high amounts of seafood and red meat; offal such as liver and kidney is particularly rich in purines. Excess consumption of purines is likely to occur on an Atkins-style diet, so if you have a family history of gout, avoid the Atkins diet.

Drinking beer or spirits is linked with an increased risk of gout, but drinking wine is not. Highly sweetened soft drinks should be avoided because they often contain large amounts of fructose, which affects the metabolism of purines and increases uric acid levels.

Purine-rich vegetables such as spinach and pulses (peas, beans, and lentils) are not generally associated with an increased risk of gout. Fruits and vegetables rich in vitamin C help the kidneys excrete uric acid. Cutting down the portion size of meat dishes is an important way of reducing gout risk, as is increasing fruit and vegetable consumption. A Mediterranean-style diet is the best way to avoid gout.

essential amino acid that is abundant in animal protein. Methionine levels are often lower in plant protein, for instance in soybeans and lentils. So if you are on a low-carb diet, you should be eating more protein from plant sources and less from animal sources. To avoid high homocysteine levels you also need an adequate intake of vitamins B_6 and B_{12} and folic acid. If you consume fewer than five daily helpings of fruits and vegetables, your folic acid intake is likely to be low, which puts you at greater risk of the harmful effects of homocysteine. A varied diet with a mixture of foods is the best bet for long-term well-being.

MYTH 4: YOU CAN'T DRINK TOO MUCH WATER

Detox diets claim to spring-clean your digestive system and help the body to dispose of toxins. Spending money on an expensive herbal "detox" supplement may encourage some people to stick to the accompanying diet, which is usually based on vegetables, fruits, and herbal teas. Avoiding processed foods and increasing fruit and vegetable consumption, in combination with stress reduction, relaxation, and regular exercise, is a regimen I cannot fault, and avoiding alcohol and coffee for two weeks certainly will do no harm.

However, I do question detox regimens that require you to drink massive amounts of water, with a total consumption of five liters a day or more. This is potentially dangerous, in both the short and the long term. Drinking such excessive amounts of water depletes the body's reserves of minerals such as sodium, potassium, calcium, magnesium, and various trace elements because of overproduction of urine. This loss of essential elements could put you at risk of collapse through a sudden fall in blood pressure or could trigger life-threatening arrhythmias (abnormal heart rhythms). In the longer term, depletion of calcium could put you at risk for osteoporosis. You will also become depleted in water-soluble vitamins such as the B vitamins, vitamin C, and folic acid. This in turn will reduce your ability to fight infection and is likely to make you lethargic, because these vitamins play a key role in energy production. If you are taking a medication that is excreted by the kidneys (most antibiotics, for example), then abnormal levels of water consumption will accelerate its elimination from your body and reduce its effectiveness. So a detox diet that involves drinking excessive amounts of water is likely to put your health at risk and should be avoided.

Advice on how much to drink each day (nonalcoholic fluids) comes from various directions. Some people seem to think that if they are thirsty for even a few moments their health is at risk. As a consequence many people are constantly drinking water or other fluids as a preventative measure. Is this a healthy thing to do? Well, there's a growing body of opinion that the likelihood of dehydration is not as high as some might think and that the risks of overhydration are not widely recognized.

Recommendations for athletes to "stay ahead of your thirst," which in practice means "drink as much fluid as possible," are now seen as bad advice. In the United States it has been recognized for some time that backpackers who collapse while hiking are more commonly overhydrated than dehydrated. A study based on blood samples taken from 488 runners at the finish line of the 2002 Boston Marathon showed that 13 percent had abnormally low sodium levels in their blood (hyponatremia). Dangerously low sodium levels can be life threatening. Investigation found that runners were drinking excessive fluids at refreshment stations because they were aiming to avoid dehydration. Most of those with the lowest blood sodium levels had drunk more than three liters (ten cups) of fluids during the race. The realization that many athletes were putting themselves at risk of hyponatremia led the U.S. Track & Field organization to introduce fresh guidelines. The new recommendations for athletes, which are just as important for casual

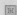
participants in sports and anybody setting off to do strenuous exercise, are: Start well hydrated (pale urine), and then drink only when thirsty. Do not drink excessive fluids.

MYTH 5: DIET IS MORE IMPORTANT THAN EXERCISE

Losing weight can be a challenge. Some people prefer the radical approach of crash diets—a week or two of severely reduced calorie intake—to shift excess weight before going on vacation or some other occasion. This can lead to the rapid loss of several pounds, but is usually followed by weight being put back on even more quickly than it was lost. This creates the so-called yo-yo effect of sudden up-and-down changes in weight. One of the main reasons for this is that when you lose weight too quickly, your metabolic rate falls. This means that you stop burning as many calories—it is your body's way of trying to make the most of the calories it has. So when you start eating normally again, more calories are stored as fat and fewer are burnt off. No matter how strictly you diet, it will become harder and harder to lose weight as your metabolic rate drops lower.

To lose weight and keep it off, it is important to reduce food intake gradually while increasing your level of exercise. Exercise helps to preserve muscle, which is one of the first things to wither on crash diets. If muscles are active, they have a higher metabolic rate, so it is easier to burn off calories. Balanced, gradual reductions in what you eat combined with progressive increases in daily levels of exercise are much more likely to leave you feeling good and produce the result you want.

On the other hand, some individuals can eat whatever they like and not gain a scrap of excess body fat. That may be because they have a very active lifestyle or simply a fast metabolic rate. Nonetheless, if they eat lots of processed and fast food and many fruits and vegetables, they are just as likely to be damaging their arteries as anyone else. They are potential candidates for heart disease. Exercise and a healthy diet are equally important for everyone.

MYTH 6: LACK OF DIETARY FIBER CAUSES COLON CANCER

For more than thirty years we have been encouraged to increase our consumption of dietary fiber to reduce the risk of colon cancer. The idea seems to have originated in an article written by Dennis Burkitt in 1969 and published in *The Lancet*. Burkitt attributed the lower level of colon cancer in African nations partly to their higher intake of dietary fiber. Nutritional advice since then has portrayed fiber as a "bowel broom," sweeping away toxins that might cause cancer and decreasing constipation in the process.

Over the years this opinion has been modified. Dietary fiber from grains and bran supplements has not led to a decrease in colon cancer. People with high fruit and vegetable intake have lower incidence of bowel cancer, but it is now believed that the micronutrients in fruits and vegetables are the protective force, rather than simply their fiber content.

Other explanations have been put forward for the increase in colon cancer in developed countries. Sugar consumption and positive energy balance (a calorie intake that exceeds what is needed for healthy living) have been strongly linked to the incidence of colon cancer. Lack of exercise, which worsens the energy balance and contributes to obesity, seems to exacerbate the problem. A high intake of red meat and meat products is also closely associated with colon cancer. Whether this is from a particular component of meat or the production of carcinogenic substances during the cooking process is not yet clear.

So the correct dietary advice for avoiding colon cancer adds up to pretty much the same as for protection from heart disease—plenty of fruits and vegetables, less red meat, and regular exercise. It is probably safe to throw out those high-bran cereals, particularly as bran can interfere with the absorption of important nutrients.

MYTH 7: PHYTOSTEROLS—a safe way to reduce cholesterol

In recent years many foods—including margarines and low-fat spreads, yogurts, drinks, and salad dressings—have been marketed with the claim that they will reduce LDL-cholesterol. These products contain plant sterols or stanols; the general name for these plant chemicals is phytosterols. The reduction in cholesterol occurs because phytosterol molecules effectively block cholesterol uptake.

These products were developed because a high level of LDL-cholesterol in the blood is a major risk factor for heart disease. A reduction in LDL-cholesterol should therefore reduce coronary heart disease. It seems to me that claims that using these products as a healthy way to lower LDL-cholesterol are premature. We do not know the long-term consequences of consuming foods that interfere with the body's cholesterol management systems. It took us many years to realize the dangers of trans fats (see page 141).

There are already areas for concern. Certainly, many of these products are low in fat but with added sugar, which is hardly ideal for good health. Some studies have shown that regular consumption of phytosterols decreases blood levels of vitamin E, beta-carotene, and lycopene. This might increase the risk of heart disease or other vascular problems. A number of investigators have found accumulation of phytosterols in the blood of some individuals and have identified these agents in atherosclerotic plaques; under these circumstances phytosterols might even be pro-atherosclerotic. Some products containing phytosterols are labeled with a recommendation not to exceed a certain intake, so consuming several such products a day may do more harm than good.

A reduction in LDL-cholesterol should reduce coronary heart disease. If this has not been demonstrated in long-term clinical trials of phytosterol-containing products, without an increased risk of other diseases, how can we be sure that they are a safe and effective approach to managing cholesterol? I will not consider consuming these products until there is proof that they are beneficial.

Remember

Always take claims for miracle diets with a pinch of salt. Diet myths often arise from a misinterpretation of the results of research. There is plenty of scope for improving long-term health through straightforward adjustments to diet and lifestyle, so pour yourself a glass of red wine and turn to the next chapter to learn about tried and tested dietary approaches to reducing heart disease and cancer.

10

SECReTS FOR PReSeRVING a HeALTHY MIND anD BODY

LIFE EXPECTANCY—and quality of life—is far more closely linked to diet and lifestyle than you might think. Over the past few decades there has been a great deal of research into the factors that distinguish societies with longer-than-average life expectancy and the risk factors for chronic disease. Yet despite an increasing body of knowledge, the global epidemic of obesity, type 2 diabetes, and related diseases is having a huge impact on the health of millions. Self-preservation is one of the strongest human instincts, but when it comes to food, despite a mass of evidence, there is frequent unwillingness to make the effort to eat well.

HOW MODERN DIET anD LIFESTYLE HaVE LOST THE PLOT

Mass production means that in industrialized countries food is cheap and readily available. Unfortunately, the processes involved can result in this food having low nutritional value. Even "fresh" fruits and vegetables are often stored for excessively long periods before we buy them, so they lose much of their vitamin content and flavor. It seems the food industry's drive for ever-increasing profits far outweighs any interest in the health of its customers, and this is at the core of many of our current health problems. Major change is necessary to improve our diet and health.

The majority of evidence for the benefits of eating healthfully points to the need to eat a varied diet with plenty of fruits and vegetables. Healthy and varied meals may take a little more time to prepare than ready-made processed food, but the effort is worth it for the more enjoyable eating experience it affords as well as for the health benefits. Sadly, in our stress-laden modern world, many people blame time pressures for avoiding this effort.

In the past, gathering together for meals was a pleasurable part of life. Nowadays, many people, young and old, eat alone, consuming poor quality food. How can healthier eating behavior be encouraged? We could start by bringing back the pleasure of the experience. Public policies on food are all about nagging and nannying. When governments talk about population-based approaches for improving health, pleasure is not usually part of the strategy. Is there an alternative approach where people will eat well because they enjoy it? Restaurants could be encouraged to provide communal tables to give single people an alternative to eating alone. This might encourage those who lack the time to shop and cook for themselves to choose healthier options than pizza delivery. But menus need to include healthier choices; many do not even offer fruit as a dessert. The Australian approach to wine in restaurants—B.Y.O. (bring your own)—might be a good way to reduce the cost of restaurant eating and allow you to drink your favorite wine at less than half the price.

Exercise is another casualty of modern life. When people spent more time walking and less time in cars, regular exercise was a part of everyday life. So perhaps it is time to rethink our urban environments. With fewer out-of-town shopping malls and more village communities we could take steps to achieving naturally healthier lifestyles.

To avoid a twenty-first-century health care disaster that no country can afford, we urgently need to change our eating habits and behavior. It is surprising how little is being done. Governments and pharmaceutical companies invest more in addressing the symptoms, for instance diabetes and heart disease, than the cause (bad diet and lack of exercise) of the problem. Tackling the root cause would be a far more effective strategy. Many people put their faith in revolutionary medicine, but there is no magic pill for diabetes or heart disease, only expensive ways of managing the illnesses.

THE POWER OF A POSITIVE MENTAL ATTITUDE

Promoting awareness of healthy lifestyles will have little effect unless an individual has the desire to change. Poor eating habits are often the result of mental attitude, depression, or lack of positive self-image. Feeling isolated and not being part of a community can add to this. In fact, many studies have concluded that depression, social isolation, and lack of social support are significant risk factors for heart disease, independent of, but of similar magnitude to, the key risk factors—smoking, high blood pressure, and high blood lipids.

The individual's role in managing his or her future disease risk is paramount. It is far more important than most of us acknowledge, especially in a society that relies on medical or surgical intervention to cure our ills. A positive attitude is known to help people recover from illness more quickly.

Coping with any sort of health problem is a drain on mental resources, but don't be afraid to seek help—getting support from others in the community was taken for granted until relatively recently. Your medical practitioner can help if you feel depressed or unable to cope. Support in your daily life can come in many forms: Talking to people with similar problems, either informally or in organized groups, works well for some; others prefer to take their mind off their anxiety by participating in different activities.

Similarly, losing weight is far easier if you are in a positive frame of mind and have support from people around you. Simple things like eating good food, having a glass of wine with your meal, and taking a daily walk can help to establish a positive attitude. And feeling optimistic means that each small step gives you a sense of making progress toward your goal of better health. Any improvement you notice reinforces this process, and it will help you set targets and achieve them.

GOOD HABITS FOR A GOOD LIFE

The message that a healthy diet and regular exercise can protect against heart disease is loud and clear. However, some people argue that it is all very well protecting yourself from heart disease, but who wants to sit out old age suffering from dementia? Recent research reveals that the factors influencing vascular health and the likelihood of heart disease are the same factors that predispose to stroke and also cause a decline in cognitive function, and possibly dementia. A diet and lifestyle that maintain vascular health—strong, flexible blood vessel walls and optimum functioning of the endothelial cells that line blood vessels (see page 29)—are therefore important throughout life.

The INTERHEART Study, published in 2004, was a milestone because it showed that 90 percent of all risk for heart attack was due to modifiable risk factors—in other words, factors that can be altered by medical treatment or by lifestyle or dietary changes. INTERHEART compared the characteristics of approximately 15,000 patients in 52 countries in order to identify the factors that placed people at risk of an acute heart attack. It concluded that the most important modifiable risks were:

- abnormal blood lipids (i.e., high cholesterol and triglycerides, particularly a high level of LDL-cholesterol with a low level of HDL-cholesterol)
- smoking

- diabetes
- high blood pressure
- obesity, particularly abdominal obesity

People who did not smoke, ate fruits and vegetables each day, exercised regularly, and habitually drank low to moderate amounts of alcohol had a very low risk of heart disease. If you could be happy living with such habits, what further motivation do you need?

An analysis of diet and lifestyle factors in relation to healthy aging of people in Europe reached similar conclusions. This study included 2,339 healthy men and women aged seventy to ninety years in 1988 to 1991, who were followed for ten years. The results showed the lowest number of deaths was in those who did not smoke, were physically active (walking, cycling, gardening), drank alcohol regularly, and had a Mediterranean diet (regular consumption of fish, pulses, vegetables, and fruits, with olive oil as the main source of fat). For those who had all these habits the likelihood of cancer and heart disease was reduced by more than two-thirds.

IT'S NEVER TOO LATE TO CHANGE

Perhaps you think it is too late to change. Think again! A number of clinical investigations into lifestyle and diet changes have shown considerable benefits in people who already have heart disease. A review of these studies was published in 2005. It found that quitting smoking reduced the number of deaths among patients with coronary heart disease by a third (in the general population death rates were halved). Increased exercise and regular alcohol consumption (one or two glasses a day) both reduced deaths by 20 to 25 percent. Dietary changes that combined increased fruits and vegetables, regular oily fish, pulses, and nuts, were estimated to almost halve the number of deaths. These figures compare favorably with studies of heart disease patients taking aspirin or statins, where deaths were reduced by 20 to 40 percent.

Regardless of drug treatment, dietary modifications can have considerable benefit. However, patients have to be willing to take the advice they are given. The longer-term effects of dietary change on 11,323 men and women who had suffered a recent heart attack were investigated in a trial in Italy. All patients were given dietary advice to increase fruits, vegetables, fish, and whole-grain products, and reduce sources of animal fat. Olive oil was to be used as much as possible, and intake of butter and other vegetable oils was to be kept to a minimum. Detailed dietary information was collected at six, eighteen, and forty-two months. The greater the compliance with the dietary advice the greater the benefit observed. Those who followed the diet most closely had only one tenth of the number of deaths of those who failed to change their diets. Clearly, if you are not personally engaged in wanting to kick out old habits, you will miss out on the benefits of making these changes.

The Lyon Diet Heart Study was designed to test the impact of a Mediterranean diet on heart disease in France. Patients in this study had already had one heart attack. Those selected for the treatment group were schooled in the changes needed for following a Mediterranean diet. They were also provided with a margarine with a composition similar to that of olive oil, enriched in alpha-linolenic acid, an essential fatty acid. After four years' follow-up the study showed a 65 percent reduction in heart problems in patients on the alpha-linolenic-rich diet. This was achieved without any change in blood cholesterol levels. Whether these benefits are exclusively due to the dietary changes is uncertain because, as mentioned in Chapter 2, a retrospective analysis of wine consumption in the Lyon Diet Heart Study showed that subjects who consumed two to four glasses of wine a day—independent of diet—had a 50 to 60 percent reduction in their likelihood of having a second heart attack. Nevertheless, these were remarkable results, as no treatment for heart disease has been able to achieve anywhere near this success. So a combination of changes in diet and moderate red wine drinking may well be the best strategy. A population-wide intervention that could reduce by half to two-thirds the level of heart attacks in patients with established coronary heart disease would save billions of dollars and increase the quality of life for millions of people.

THE KEY TO HEALTHY MEDITERRANEAN LIVING

The concept of using a Mediterranean-style diet to reduce the incidence of heart disease originated from the Seven Countries Study. This study was started in the 1950s by American nutritionist Dr. Ancel Keys. After fifteen years there was clear evidence in Crete of a significantly lower number of deaths from heart disease. Also, for a given blood pressure or cholesterol level, there was much lower risk of heart attack. This suggested the existence of a number of protective factors.

The Cretan Mediterranean diet was high in fruits, vegetables, fish, pulses, whole-grain foods and nuts—and was therefore rich in vitamins and minerals, with ample sources of plant protein—and low in meat, refined starch, and sugar. It was also relatively high in fat—up to 35 percent of calorie intake was from fat—but this was mainly monounsaturated fat from olive oil.

The Seven Countries Study correlated the low level of heart disease with a reduced level of saturated fat and increased level of monounsaturated fat in the Cretan diet, and it became the model for the recommendation that a Mediterranean diet was best for heart health. However, many nutritionists and government advisers failed to convert the evidence into suitable dietary recommendations. Instead of recommending that saturated fat consumption be reduced while increasing the intake of monounsaturated fat to 20 to 25 percent of calorie intake, the message was spread that all fat is harmful; so everybody was encouraged to reduce their fat intake as much as possible. This was the biggest error in judgment the nutrition world has ever made. Only relatively recently has the consumption of olive oil been widely advocated. There is now a growing awareness that monounsaturated and polyunsaturated fats actually improve health. The dietary recommendations of this book focus on the key elements of a healthy Mediterranean diet.

SECRETS OF THE CRETAN DIET

The Cretan way of eating held other nutritional secrets, which we now appreciate contribute to a lower risk of heart disease. A study in 2001 reviewed the beneficial components of the Cretan diet. One of the most important differences compared to other diets was the relative abundance of omega-3 polyunsaturated fatty acids (PUFAs).

There were diverse sources of omega-3 PUFAs in the Cretan diet in the 1960s. Perhaps the most important of these was purslane, a common wild plant. It does not contain particularly high amounts of fatty acids but typically has four to five times more omega-3 than omega-6 PUFAs. It has a slightly peppery flavor and is used in salads and soups. However, eating purslane was not the Cretans' main dietary source of omega-3 PUFAs. Other animals were also eating it, thereby producing foods naturally high in omega-3 PUFAs. Chickens laid eggs with a healthy ratio of PUFAs, whereas most of the eggs we buy, from corn-fed chickens, have an unhealthy 20 to 1 ratio of omega-6 to omega-3 PUFAs. Similarly, although meat-based meals were rare, the meat was naturally high in omega-3 PUFAs. Cheese and yogurt were also better as a result of the natural diet of the animals. Even snails, which were a popular dish in Crete, were rich in omega-3 PUFAs.

Walnuts, abundant in Crete, are another rich source of omega-3 PUFAs. Figs grow easily in Crete and are eaten both fresh and dried; they have only traces of fat, but this, too, is healthy fat. Olive oil is rich in monounsaturated oleic acid and has low amounts of omega-6 PUFAs. No wonder the traditional Cretan diet had a healthy mix of PUFAs.

Today, the majority of us do not get enough omega-3 PUFAs. Since we have been encouraged to replace saturated fats with polyunsaturated fats, the general recommendation has been to consume vegetable oils such as sunflower, safflower, and corn oils. But these are all rich in omega-6 PUFAs and contain little if any omega-3 PUFAs. The ideal ratio of omega-6 to omega-3 PUFAs is considered to be somewhere between 2 to 1 and 1 to 1. Since the "polyunsaturated fats are best" message has taken root, most people consume at least ten to fifteen times more omega-6 PUFAs than omega-3. This is creating an unhealthy imbalance, which interferes with the body's ability to metabolize omega-3 PUFAs from plant sources to EPA (eicosapentaenoic acid) and DHA (docosahexaenoic acid), which the brain and other tissues need for optimal health. Some of the recommended recipes in this book are designed to correct the imbalance found in most modern diets.

NUTS TO CRACK CHOLESTEROL

As mentioned in Chapter 4, the Adventist Health Study—a large-scale survey in California—found clear evidence that people who consume nuts regularly have a decreased risk of coronary heart disease.

Walnuts have been singled out for study because they are a particularly rich source of healthy omega-3 polyunsaturated fats. Clinical investigations have shown that daily walnut consumption can improve the blood lipid profiles of men and women (abnormal blood lipids are a key risk factor for heart disease). In a study in Spain, patients with raised cholesterol ate 40 to 50 grams (about 1.5 to 1.75 ounces) of walnuts every day for six weeks. Their LDL-cholesterol (bad cholesterol) dropped by an average of 6 percent. HDL-cholesterol (good cholesterol) did not change, thus the ratio of HDL- to LDL-cholesterol was improved, which is an additional benefit. Similar improvements were seen in a study of diabetic patients who ate 30 grams (about 1 ounce) of walnuts a day for six months. Their LDL-cholesterol decreased by 10 percent and their HDL-cholesterol ratio also improved. These changes may sound small, but they are enough to have an effect on the risk of heart disease.

The U.S. Food and Drug Administration permits a qualified recommendation that 1.5 ounces of walnuts a day may reduce coronary heart disease. For maximum benefit, the walnuts should be used to replace other foods with an equivalent number of calories, particularly foods high in saturated fats. Almonds and most other nuts are high in healthy monounsaturated fats, but they also contain omega-6 PUFAs and less omega-3. Omega-6 PUFAs reduce both LDL- and HDL-cholesterol: A reduction in HDL-cholesterol can be seen as a disadvantage. However, nuts also provide valuable minerals (see Chapter 11), and there is a case for eating a variety of nuts as substitutes for other sources of fat and protein in the diet, such as meat.

LOWER WEIGHT EQUALS BETTER HEALTH

Many people experience an expanding waistline as they grow older; a middle-age spread is considered perfectly normal. But the more weight you gain from your late twenties to your fifties the greater your risk of heart disease, diabetes, and cancer. However, if you are already "well covered" in your early twenties and don't put on much weight as you get older, then the risk of these diseases does not increase as much as it does for somebody who gains a lot of weight over this time. It seems that slight overeating—regularly consuming more calories than your body needs, resulting in a positive energy balance—could be the trigger for diabetes. It is also thought that raised levels of insulin associated with excess calorie intake may drive the growth of cancerous cells.

DIETS THAT IMPROVE BLOOD PRESSURE

Increased girth seems to have a particular influence on blood pressure. If you have slightly raised blood pressure (between 120/80 and 140/90 mmHg), and are at the borderline of needing to take a prescription medicine, weight loss is one of the best ways to bring blood pressure down. Even if you are already taking prescription medications for high blood pressure, weight loss can help by making the treatment more effective. For every two pounds lost, blood pressure drops by about 1 mmHg. That may not sound a lot, but if you lose ten to twenty pounds, it will make a real difference to your long-term well-being, because high blood pressure is a major risk factor for heart disease. A reduced calorie intake combined with regular aerobic exercise has the greatest benefits.

A study in Oxfordshire, England, showed that simply eating more fruits and vegetables can reduce blood pressure. Participants were encouraged to eat at least five portions of fruits and vegetables a day. After six months blood pressure showed similar decreases to those reported for the DASH Diet (see page 161). The increased intake of vitamins, minerals, and other micronutrients will also decrease the risk of heart disease over the longer term.

The INTERMAP Study investigated dietary factors influencing blood pressure in 4,680 men and women aged from forty to fifty-nine years in Japan, China, the United Kingdom, and the United States. It identified a link between increased consumption of plant protein and reduced blood pressure. A further study in China went on to test the effect of consuming 40 grams (about 1.5 ounces) of soy protein a day for twelve weeks. It found that soy protein reduced blood pressure by an average of 4 mmHg compared to those eating the control diet.

MACRONUTRIENTS, HEART DISEASE, AND WEIGHT LOSS

The conclusions from the DASH Diet have been extended through the Optimal MacroNutrient Intake Trial to Prevent Heart Disease (OmniHeart)

A number of studies have attempted to define the ideal diet for people who are overweight and have high blood pressure. The best results have been obtained with a combination of lifestyle changes and the Dietary Approaches to Stop Hypertension (DASH) Diet. The DASH Diet aims for an increase in fruits and vegetables (nine to twelve servings a day), a switch from full-fat to low-fat dairy products, and an overall reduction in the intake of saturated fat and total fat. In a clinical trial at four American medical centers, participants with a Body Mass Index of 25 or more (20 to 25 is considered normal—see tables on pages 278 and 279) were set a weight loss target of 15 pounds in six months. They were asked to exercise at moderate intensity for 180 minutes per week, reduce dietary salt, and restrict alcohol intake to two drinks a day for men (one for women). For those following this regimen the average decrease in blood pressure was 11 mmHg. In the study only 34 percent met their weight loss goals. However, only 13 percent reduced their salt intake to the desired level, and only 27 percent increased fruit and vegetable consumption to the required amount—it seems likely that the benefits of this diet would be much greater if more participants were able to meet the targets.

Study. This investigated how different percentages of macronutrients (i.e., carbohydrate, fat, and protein) altered the response to the DASH Diet. Three diets were compared:

- High carbohydrate (58 percent of calories from carbohydrate, 27 percent from fat, 15 percent from protein)
- High fat (48 percent of calories from carbohydrate, 37 percent from fat, 15 percent from protein)
- High protein (48 percent of calories from carbohydrate, 27 percent from fat, 25 percent from protein)

All the diets followed the DASH approach of high fruit and vegetable consumption, low saturated fat, and low salt. The high-fat diet was achieved by increasing monounsaturated fat through the use of vegetable oils (olive, canola, and safflower) combined with increased amounts of nuts and seeds. Two-thirds of the increased protein intake in the high-protein diet was from plant sources (pulses, grains, nuts, and seeds). The selection of foods and drinks on the DASH Diet also reduces sugar consumption.

The study participants were mainly overweight (34 percent) or obese (45 percent). Since losing weight will itself affect blood pressure, the individuals' diets were designed to maintain their existing body weight and provide the same number of calories. Every participant followed each diet for a period of six weeks, with the diets being allocated in a random order.

All diets led to reduced blood pressure and lowered LDL-cholesterol; the high-carbohydrate diet had least effect. The high-protein diet reduced LDL-cholesterol more than the other diets, but it also reduced HDL-cholesterol, which is an unwanted effect. The high-fat diet was most favorable for maintaining or increasing HDL-cholesterol. High-carbohydrate diets raised blood triglyceride levels, whereas triglycerides were reduced by the high-fat diet, and to an even greater extent by the high-protein diet.

The reduction in blood pressure on these diets is explained by the lower salt (sodium) consumption and higher potassium consumption from eating more fruits and vegetables. Eating whole-grain foods and low-fat dairy products increases magnesium and calcium intake, which also favors lower blood pressure.

Based on observed changes in blood pressure and blood lipids, the ten-year risk of coronary heart disease was calculated for each diet. The high-protein and high-fat diets were better than the high-carbohydrate diet. The best diet would seem to be a fusion of the high-fat and high-protein diets: not more than 50 percent of calories from carbohydrate, approximately 30 percent from fat (of which at least half is monounsaturated fat), and 20 percent from protein. Adopting this type of diet together with small reductions in calorie intake is likely to improve health and lead to a gradual reduction in weight.

It is interesting to note that 10 percent of the subjects on the high-protein diet in the OmniHeart Study reported a loss of appetite; this might make it easier to lose weight on a high-protein diet. Increasing the proportion of calories from protein to around 25 percent may be helpful when attempting to lose weight. However, in the long term a high-protein diet is likely to reduce HDL-cholesterol, which is not a desirable goal.

LIFESTYLE CHOICES THAT HELP PREVENT CANCER

Most people know that obesity increases the risk of diabetes. But do they realize that obesity can almost double their chance of developing cancer? The link between obesity and cancer is not simply a matter of being overweight. Excess calorie intake can cause elevated levels of the hormone insulin, and this may promote the growth of cancerous cells. In addition, foods that cause obesity are generally unhealthy and lack nutrients that can help protect against cancer.

Considerable evidence suggests that diet is a key factor influencing the likelihood of cancer. The finger of blame points to certain dietary habits that cause harm. But the key question, which remains largely unanswered, is which dietary factors provide protection from cancer?

In 1997 a World Cancer Research Fund report concluded that 30 to 40 percent of all cancers could be prevented by following certain diet guidelines, getting regular exercise, and avoiding being overweight. The diet and lifestyle recommendations are basically the same as those I suggest: a nutritionally balanced diet with increased consumption of foods of plant origin and less meat. Excess alcohol consumption was discouraged because of its links to breast, colon, liver, mouth, and throat cancers. As discussed elsewhere, moderate wine drinkers often have low levels of cancer. The risk of cancer from alcohol is increased if other aspects of nutrition are poor. For example, it is known that alcohol interferes with the absorption of folic acid. All alcohol drinkers should make sure their diets are rich in fruits and vegetables to reduce the likelihood of cancer.

The factors leading to tumor growth and spread are still poorly understood. Should we be boosting our natural defense systems so the body is more successful in eliminating cancerous cells when they first appear? Data gathered from patients taking immunosuppressive drugs, for instance after a kidney transplant, show an increased prevalence of tumors. This indicates that the immune system plays a constant role in checking the growth of tumors—so-called immune surveillance. To decrease the risk of cancer, and indeed infection, it is important to keep your immune system functioning well through good nutrition. Aging is associated with a decline in immune function—another reason why a healthy diet that protects the immune system is even more important as we get older.

Certain foods are said to reduce cancer risk, but it is often hard to pinpoint the specific components that are important. A four-year investigation into the relationship between levels of vitamin C in the blood and risk of heart disease and cancer studied 19,496 men and women aged forty-five to seventy-nine years. In both men and women the lower the vitamin C levels the greater the likelihood of heart disease. In men this was also true for cancer. Subjects with the lowest vitamin C levels were eating no more than two portions of fruits and vegetables a day. In this study the contribution from other nutrients besides vitamin C was not examined.

High tomato consumption in Italy and other Mediterranean countries has been linked to much lower levels of prostate cancer and less frequent cancer of the lung, breast, ovary, and colon. This is often attributed to the protective effects of lycopene, a carotenoid that is abundant in tomatoes. But in Mediterranean countries tomatoes are often served or cooked with olive oil as part of a generally healthy eating pattern, and it is difficult to distinguish the effects of this specific nutrient. The link to lycopene is not yet sufficiently strong to state that it is responsible for preventing prostate cancer. I do not advocate lycopene supplements as an alternative to healthy eating. Besides tomatoes—and this includes canned, dried and puréed tomatoes—other natural sources of lycopene include watermelon, pink grapefruit, guava, and papaya.

Deficiencies in the trace element selenium have been linked to cancer in some countries. Selenium is essential for thyroid hormone production, and the immune system is dependent on adequate selenium intake. Selenium deficiency is associated with an increased risk of several cancers, including prostate, lung, breast, and colon. It is also considered to increase the likelihood of atherosclerosis, arthritis, accelerated aging, and a number of brain diseases. In most countries selenium intake is thought to be adequate in people with a varied healthy diet because most fruits, vegetables, and animal food products contain some selenium. But in areas of selenium-deficient soil the whole spectrum of foods can be low in selenium. The soil in the northwest and northeast areas of the United States, Britain, and other European countries are relatively selenium deficient. The number of people bordering on deficiency may be greater than thought. Boosting dietary sources of selenium by eating more seafood—or one or two Brazil nuts a day—may therefore be beneficial. Be aware, however, that selenium can be toxic in high doses.

How much do food production techniques contribute to cancer? Unnatural additions to food may result from pesticide residues or chemicals that are added to foods during manufacturing and processing in order to preserve food and prolong storage times, as well as for flavoring, sweetening, and coloring. The effect of these chemical additives on our health is difficult to evaluate. Studies of eating habits tend to group together types of food irrespective of their manufacture and quality. I think the best way to avoid any possible health problems associated with food additives is to eat fresh, natural, organic food as much as possible. Steer clear of manufactured foods where the ingredient list looks like something from a chemistry set rather than a recipe book.

Sometimes additives are used in winemaking as well. There are a number of authorized chemicals that can be used, for instance, to boost yeast function, but apart from sulphites I do not think I have ever seen any additives declared; I think this information would be helpful to consumers. Even organic wines may not be free of additives, because organic status generally refers to the grape growing rather than the winemaking.

Cooking itself can be a source of toxic, potentially cancer-causing chemicals. For instance, cooking with oils containing polyunsaturated fats generates a mixture of reactive compounds that may increase the risk of cancer or heart disease. High-temperature cooking—broiling, roasting, and particularly barbecuing—is another source of many potentially toxic chemicals. However, it seems likely that these cooking techniques do not present major risks to health if you use them only occasionally. The danger from carcinogens in barbecued food is of concern only if you eat this type of food every day. Cooking food without charring is a good starting point. Overcooking food can also destroy vitamins and other nutrients.

THE IMPORTANCE OF VITAMIN D

Vitamin D plays a crucial role in stimulating intestinal absorption of calcium, without which bone strength can be compromised, eventually leading to osteoporosis. Vitamin D also reduces the likelihood of breast, lung, colon, and prostate cancer, because it inhibits the growth of cancer cells. Low vitamin D make levels high blood pressure more likely, and are associated with an increased risk of heart disease. Vitamin D deficiency has also been linked to autoimmune diseases such as rheumatoid arthritis and multiple sclerosis.

Exposure to the sun is a key source of vitamin D—UV light stimulates vitamin D production in the skin. In recent decades many people have become fearful of sun exposure because of the risk of skin cancer; using sunscreen cuts out a large percentage of UV sunlight. Despite concerns about skin cancer, it is not healthy to avoid all skin exposure to sunlight. Getting the balance right means regular exposure to sunlight, but only for short periods and, above all, avoiding sunburn. Dark-skinned people living in northern latitudes are most likely to be vitamin D deficient, because with low sun exposure very little UV light penetrates darker skin to stimulate vitamin D synthesis. Vitamin D status frequently gets worse as people get older and are less likely to expose their skin to sunlight. Vitamin D synthesized in skin is stored in fat, but this is not sufficient to maintain vitamin D levels throughout the year.

Eating oily fish is a good way to maintain vitamin D levels. Apart from oily fish, very few foods naturally contain enough vitamin D to meet our daily needs. Vitamin D fortification of many foods (e.g., breakfast cereals and dairy products) is common in the United States and Europe.

AVOIDING OSTEOPOROSIS

What is important for preventing osteoporosis? Well, actually it reads like a checklist for good cardiovascular health: adequate vitamin D, plenty of fruits and green vegetables, a good balance of minerals—calcium being the most important, but by no means the only one—and plenty of exercise!

Bone mass is greatest between twenty-five and forty years of age in both men and women. After this, loss of bone density and bone strength occur progressively with age. Osteoporosis is the condition in which bone structure is modified and weakened to such an extent that there is a risk of bone fractures. It affects one in three women and one in twelve men and is more common in people with risk factors for heart disease.

Most people are surprised to learn that bone is a very dynamic structure; it is constantly being broken down and rebuilt so that old bone is replaced by new bone. This cycle is balanced by the relationship between cells that form bone (osteoblasts) and cells that break it down (osteoclasts). As we get older it seems that osteoclast activity increases at a greater rate than osteoblast, so that bone density decreases.

A variety of hormones, together with certain dietary vitamins and minerals, influence this balance of bone breakdown and renewal. For women, considerable emphasis is given to the benefits of estrogen for maintaining bone strength. The decline in estrogen levels after menopause is often cited as a major risk factor for osteoporosis. But the weightlessness experienced by astronauts during space flights also leads to a small but rapid decrease in bone mass. I mention this simply to emphasize the complex issues of how bone strength is maintained and the fact that we don't yet know all the answers when it comes to optimizing bone strength.

Many people think that their best defense against osteoporosis is to make sure they consume plenty of dairy products, which are a rich source of calcium. There is no doubt that adequate calcium is required throughout life to maintain optimal bone strength, but this alone is not sufficient to prevent osteoporosis. In the Nurses' Health Study a lower risk of hip fracture was observed in those with an adequate intake of vitamin D. There was no relationship between milk consumption and the occurrence of hip fractures. Other analyses have often failed to show that calcium intake is related to fracture risk, except when there is evidence of very low calcium intake.

A healthy diet generally has an adequate intake of both calcium and vitamin D, but other vitamins and micronutrients are also important for maximum bone strength. Vitamin K, a fat-soluble vitamin, plays a critical role in bone formation. Green leafy vegetables are a rich source of vitamin K, yet some writers warn about oxalates (naturally occurring plant chemicals found in some green vegetables) interfering with calcium absorption, as though green vegetables might promote osteoporosis! Vitamin C is essential for the production of collagen (part of the structure of bones and connective tissue)—fresh fruit is one of the richest sources of vitamin C.

Diets high in salt (sodium chloride) and low in potassium promote calcium loss by excretion through the kidneys. Reducing salt intake and eating more fruit will help prevent this so that the most efficient use of calcium from all food sources is achieved. Adequate magnesium is a prerequisite for the formation of strong, healthy bones. Intakes of several other minerals and trace elements—boron, copper, fluoride, manganese, silicon, and zinc—are important for good bone strength. These are all linked to greater bone mineral density, but their respective importance in preventing osteoporosis has yet to be fully evaluated. There seems no doubt that a varied diet, with plenty of fruits and vegetables, is the best way to satisfy the nutritional needs for bone health.

Although fluoride plays a key role in bone development, excess fluoride intake can reduce bone quality and may increase fracture risk. So fluoride supplements should be avoided. Most diets usually provide sufficient fluoride, either through the water supply or from vegetables.

Supplements containing excess amounts of vitamin A in the form of retinol, the antiaging vitamin for skin, also promote bone weakening and have been linked to a two-fold increase in hip fractures. Taking more than 1,500 micrograms a day is harmful, so if you take more than one supplement, you should work out whether you exceed this amount.

Another key factor for maximum bone strength is regular physical exercise, particularly load-bearing, or weight-bearing, exercise. Essentially this means walking, running, and other activities that use the weight of the body rather than exercises done while lying on the floor or swimming. Serious shopping, carrying heavy bags around for several hours, could be considered good exercise!

The genetic influences on osteoporosis are not yet understood. If you know that you have a family history of this problem, it makes sense to make an extra effort to follow a diet and exercise program that will reduce your risk.

BEATING THE METABOLIC CLOCK—WHEN TO EAT

Many weight-loss diets are prescriptive about the number of calories to eat at different times of the day. Most recommend breakfast as a key meal. Others discourage eating most of your calories in the evening—in other words, dinner as a main meal is considered unhealthy. The evidence to support these ideas is weak. In many European countries, particularly in wine-drinking areas, it is common to eat the main meal in the evening, accompanied by wine. Lunch may be lighter, but is often also accompanied by wine (and sometimes followed by a siesta). Breakfast is often a minimal affair. Why, then, is breakfast so strongly advocated elsewhere?

It will not surprise readers to know that my main meal generally is dinner, complemented with wine. I rarely eat much for breakfast because I tend not to feel hungry early in the morning. Clearly, if you have a very active lifestyle, then you probably need to eat more for breakfast. But even when I worked on my parents' dairy farm with a 6 a.m. start, I preferred to eat breakfast around 10 a.m., after I had done the morning milking. So skipping an early breakfast and substituting it with brunch or an early lunch may suit some people.

Many diets encourage snacks between meals. The reasons put forward include boosting the metabolism to make it more efficient and keeping energy levels topped up to prevent overeating at the next meal. In fact, some degree of fasting between meals is a good idea: It helps to burn fat and improve the function of the endothelial cells that line our blood vessels. Carbohydrate-rich snacks are the worse choice, as they stop your body from moving into fat-burning mode. If you find you need to eat snacks, then fruits and raw vegetables are the best option.

Eating meals slowly is a good way to avoid overeating. Most countries around the Mediterranean traditionally favor extended mealtimes, often made up of a number of small courses; these give the best opportunity to satisfy the appetite without eating too much. An aperitif such as a small glass of wine with a few olives or nuts (unsalted, and not honey roasted) may also help to limit the total amount you eat. Eat less, but enjoy it more!

Individuals differ in what suits them. I think everybody needs to work out the mealtimes that best meet their energy needs and satisfy their hunger. A regular pattern of eating is certainly a good idea so that your body adapts to a routine. The bottom line is that if your calorie count regularly exceeds your metabolic needs over twenty-four hours, then you will start to put on weight.

A GOOD NIGHT'S SLEEP

Sleep patterns can affect appetite and metabolic activity, which can influence overeating. Lack of sleep can lead to overeating the wrong foods. A study of the effects of sleep deprivation on healthy volunteers found that sleep restriction resulted in hormonal changes and altered appetite. Not only were the volunteers hungrier, but they also wanted to consume more carbohydrate-rich food. So a hearty breakfast after a poor night's sleep is probably not a good idea—you may feel ravenously hungry, but you will consume more calories than your body needs.

Another study of healthy subjects confirmed that sleep deprivation activates the stress hormones cortisol and noradrenaline, which stimulate your body to produce glucose. This in turn can create a state of impaired glucose tolerance—the prediabetic state.

The risk of diabetes is real. A two- to three-fold increase in diabetes has been reported in Japanese patients with poor sleep patterns. This is in agreement with an American analysis of fasting glucose and glucose tolerance tests on 1,486 subjects aged fifty-three to ninety-three. People enrolled in this study also filled out a questionnaire about their sleep patterns. Of these people, almost 21 percent had diabetes, and a further 28 percent had impaired glucose tolerance. People sleeping less than five hours were two and a half times more likely to have diabetes than those sleeping seven to eight hours. Interestingly, those sleeping nine hours or more were also twice as likely to suffer from diabetes and impaired glucose tolerance.

My best advice is to get enough sleep, but don't have too many long lie-ins. And resist those early starts for breakfast meetings, not just for your sanity, but also to protect you from obesity and diabetes.

DAILY EXERCISE—WHY DO IT?

Our bodies are designed for exercise, but nowadays our daily lives require us to do less and less; many people go through the day without doing any exercise at all! But for effective weight loss and to protect overall health, exercise is vital. It is crucial for providing the right balance between calorie consumption and energy expenditure.

As a seven-year-old living in the countryside, I cycled two miles to school each morning. From the age of ten, with a change of school, this increased to five miles each way. This was not unusual for my peer group—although admittedly country roads were much quieter forty years ago. These days many children don't walk or cycle to school and some don't play sports, either. This lack of exercise is putting many children at risk of premature heart disease and diabetes. It also establishes a pattern that is harder to break in adulthood. Heart disease in your sixties or seventies can severely reduce quality of life. Heart disease in your thirties or forties will lead to many lost years.

The speed at which our bodies burn calories while resting is called the basal metabolic rate (BMR). This is influenced by our hormonal systems. Regular exercise stimulates muscle activity and this can increase our BMR because muscle cells are metabolically more active than other body cells— even when they are resting. As we get older, our metabolic rate decreases. Fewer calories are therefore required to meet energy needs—and any excess consumption accumulates as body fat. Doing less exercise as you get older makes this worse. Breaking this cycle by eating less and becoming more active are key goals for anybody trying to manage their weight.

Physical activity lowers blood pressure, increases insulin sensitivity, and improves blood lipid levels and blood vessel health. Exercising before eating improves vascular function after the meal—when fat is digested and absorbed, smaller increases in LDL-cholesterol and triglyceride levels have been observed in both lean and obese individuals.

People who do not engage in any physical activity are increasing their risk of both heart disease and diabetes. They are also more likely to develop cancer. Exercise is essential for losing visceral (abdominal) fat, which is important for preventing diabetes. Diet alone does not easily achieve this. If you are overweight and have impaired glucose tolerance, a combination of exercise and a change of diet can bring you back from the brink of diabetes. This is true for every age group, from children to the elderly. If you have already had a heart attack, daily moderate exercise is more successful than any medical treatment for preventing heart failure. It reduces hospitalization and greatly improves overall quality of life.

You don't have to be a marathon runner for exercise to make you feel good. It may be exhausting at first, but starting an exercise program will bring greater energy. Regular fairly strenuous exercise helps create a positive self-image. It is an effective form of stress relief and increases self-confidence. In fact, exercise programs often work well as an alternative prescription for treating people with depression.

What sort of exercise? To gain the maximum benefit, an hour a day is thought to be best. But this does not need to be sixty minutes of strenuous exercise in the gym or pounding the streets until your joints suffer damage. In fact, suddenly adopting a very vigorous program of exercise can increase the likelihood of thrombosis. A recent study of healthy male volunteers found that short-term vigorous exercise increased the risk of blood clotting. However, thirty minutes of exercise at sixty percent of maximum effort five days a week for eight weeks resulted in a measurably reduced risk of blood clotting, both at rest and during exercise. The volunteers then stopped this schedule of exercising. Eight weeks later the beneficial effects of their training were lost. This emphasizes the need for sustaining a regular pattern of exercise.

A brisk walk is a good starting point. Introduce exercise into your day by parking your car a fifteen- to thirty-minute walk from where you work, or if you use public transportation, take it to a different location that requires you to walk the final mile (or two) to work. You might prefer to take a walk when you leave work in the evening or at lunchtime. Variety is a good idea; otherwise your daily walk may become a chore. So if possible, change your route or destination. While you walk, observe what is going on around you—the changing seasons, interesting buildings, other people. But most important, enjoy doing it.

Whatever you decide to do, you should start off small and gradually increase the amount you do each day. It's not necessary to join a gym to get an hour of moderate exercise a day. A brisk walk to the store, particularly if it involves an uphill section, or using the stairs rather than the elevator, may represent a cardiovascular workout as good as going to the gym, but with the added bonus (if you are in the right environment) of being in fresh air.

For people living at higher altitudes (3,300 feet or more), the additional physical effort involved in simple daily routines may explain why longevity is greatest in mountain regions.

REDUCING THE RISK OF DEMENTIA

A healthy mind requires a healthy body. All the risk factors for heart disease (high blood pressure, high LDL-cholesterol, smoking, diabetes, high homocysteine levels) have been linked to impaired cognitive function. Some studies have shown an even closer association in patients with peripheral artery disease. All these observations point to the need to keep blood vessels healthy to keep the brain at top form.

As mentioned in Chapter 2, studies of red wine drinkers show a lower level of dementia. This may reflect the beneficial actions of procyanidins on blood vessel function in the brain.

Keeping the brain active is equally important. Magnetic resonance imaging (MRI) can reveal which parts of the brain are involved in different tasks. MRI shows this by measuring vasodilation in particular brain areas, reflecting the increase in metabolic activity. Retaining the ability of each part of the brain to trigger vasodilation in response to increased brain activity is critical, because this responsiveness allows the blood supply to increase the availability of nutrients to the brain. Performing different types of mental activity uses different areas of the brain.

Exercise also appears to play an important part in preventing mental decline. The FINE (Finland, Italy, and the Netherlands Elderly) Study examined the mental ability of elderly men and related it to their level of exercise over fifteen years. Comparisons showed that reduced mental ability was closely associated with a decrease in physical activity (walking, gardening, cycling, and other sporting activities). Those who maintained or increased their physical activity had the best mental ability. In the United States, a study of 2,300 men aged seventy-one to ninety-three years found that dementia was twice as likely in men who walked the least compared to those walking two or more miles a day. Similar results were found for women in the Nurses' Health Study. It is still uncertain whether there is a direct link between cardiovascular fitness and brain function. It may be that different types of physical exercise increase activity in different parts of the brain, keeping manual dextcrity, hand-to-eye coordination, and balance in better shape. This in turn may help maintain various other abilities.

PROTECTING YOUR EYESIGHT

Cataracts and age-related macular degeneration are the most common reasons for poor vision and blindness in old age. A cataract is cloudiness in the lens of the eye, which leads to blurred or poor vision, particularly in low light. Cataracts can be removed surgically in a simple operation. Macular degeneration is a much greater problem because there are not yet any proven treatments. Macular degeneration leads to permanent vision loss, so a lifelong appreciation of the need to look after your eyesight is important.

The macula is the central area of the retina at the back of the eye. It is the area of the retina responsible for the sharpest vision. In the center of the macula there is a small indentation called the fovea. The fovea consists of mainly cone cells, which detect different colored light depending on their light sensitivity (red, green/yellow, or blue). If the function of these cells deteriorates, they lose their ability to detect light. Damage to the macula leads to blurred or distorted vision and eventually blind spots. This can prevent you from driving and makes reading difficult.

There are two types of macular degeneration: dry and wet. The dry type, in which loss of vision occurs gradually, is more common. The wet type of macular degeneration is a much more severe problem, which can rapidly lead to blindness. New blood vessels grow under the macula and then start to bleed or leak. Laser treatment can be used to stop the bleeding, but this itself can cause retinal damage and lead to further vision loss. And it does not eliminate the problem, so rapid worsening of vision still may occur.

What are the most important factors that put people at risk of macular degeneration? You cannot change your age or family history; women are more likely to be affected than men; and Caucasians have a higher risk than people of other ethnic origins. Quitting smoking is the best thing you can do to avoid macular degeneration. Excess exposure to strong light may contribute to retinal damage. People with coronary heart disease are more likely to suffer from macular degeneration, so any steps you take to avoid heart disease, such as reducing high cholesterol levels and high blood pressure, are likely to help. If you do not protect the health of your blood vessels, then the retina, like many other vital organs, is going to suffer.

Can the carrot help you avoid the stick? As well as making sure your diet and lifestyle are as heart-healthy as possible, certain nutrients play a specific role in maintaining eye health. The full name for the macula is *macula lutea*, which means "yellow spot" (from Latin—*luteus*, yellow; *macula*, spot). The yellow color of the macula is due to a high concentration of carotenoids in macular tissue. Carotenoids in the macula are thought to serve two functions: They protect the retinal cells by absorbing UV light and blue light, which are the most damaging wavelengths, and they act as antioxidants by neutralizing free radicals generated by excessive exposure of the eye to light. So carotenoids function as a sort of natural sunscreen for the retina. They are also reported to improve sensitivity to light contrasts and color perception. So there is some truth in the tale that carrots will help you see in the dark. The key carotenoids are lutein and zeaxanthin. The macula cells absorb these carotenoids from the blood and selectively concentrate them to form this pigment screen, which is why lutein and zeaxanthin are thought to be absolutely critical for good eye health.

People with low levels of these carotenoids in the retina are more likely to suffer from poor vision and blindness, so what you eat plays an important part in protecting your eyesight. A number of foods are rich in lutein and zeaxanthin; green vegetables such as spinach, green cabbage, broccoli, and kale are excellent sources of these carotenoids. Sweet potatoes, corn, peas, green beans, and oranges are also good sources. Carrots have some of these carotenoids, but they are not the best source. These carotenoids are best absorbed when eaten with meals that contain fat. This means it is better to eat salads with an olive oil–based vinaigrette rather than a low-fat salad dressing.

Other nutrients also affect eye health. For instance, adequate consumption of omega-3 fatty acids is essential for optimal function of the retina. Procyanidins may also be useful through their effects on blood vessel function. The procyanidin extract from pine bark called pycnogenol has been reported to have some beneficial effects in treating diabetic retinopathy, which bears some similarity to the wet type of age-related macular degeneration. The best diet to prevent macular degeneration most likely is a Mediterranean diet rich in green vegetables, with a daily glass of procyanidin-rich wine.

YOUR DENTIST WILL SEE YOU NOW

You may be surprised to learn that regular dental checkups can play an important part in preventing heart disease. Poor gum health and dental infections can increase the risk of heart attacks and stroke. It is too easy to put off a visit to the dentist because an occasional bleeding gum is not a symptom to be concerned about, or a painful tooth might seem trivial.

These small infections are a drip-by-drip infusion of toxins into the blood, which can cause inflammation in your blood vessels. This may make atherosclerosis more severe, or worse, trigger a blood clot to form. If your body is not working flat out to eliminate any blood clot as it forms, this may cause a heart attack or stroke. It makes sense to avoid this by visiting your dentist every six months.

SUPPLEMENTS—NO SUBSTITUTE FOR A HEALTHY DIET

People who eat more fruits and vegetables are less likely to suffer from heart disease and cancer. Although we understand the importance of having recommended daily amounts of a number of vitamins, clinical trials to correct dietary deficiencies of particular vitamins or minerals with supplements have been a dismal failure. Despite this, advice to take supplements is widespread. Health journalists in magazines and on radio and television often advocate specific products. Most of this advice is based on the premise that dietary gaps in specific nutrients can be replaced through supplements. Generally these recommendations appear highly logical, but when tested in clinical trials the supplements either have conferred no benefit or have proved to be more harmful than not taking them at all. It is important to understand that a good diet should—with very few exceptions—not need supplements, and supplements are not an alternative to a good diet.

Why supplements work less well than might be expected is a difficult question to answer. It may be because some supplements contain contaminants arising from the manufacturing process that counteract the benefits. Even "natural" products may suffer from the processes of manufacture into a convenient tablet or capsule. The multibillion-dollar vitamin and mineral supplement market has so far not been as closely regulated as the pharmaceutical industry. My own analyses of herbal remedies such as grape seed, hawthorn, and cranberry products show tremendous variation in quality; many of them deserve to be banned.

In Europe new legislation was introduced in 2005 to regulate supplements and alternative remedies. The U.S. Food and Drug Administration is also examining how to exert greater control over these products. Despite the outcry of certain consumers and lobby groups who do not want increased regulation, the intention is to protect the users of these products. Legislation has two main aims: to improve quality and safety, and to prevent misleading claims for the benefits of a product. This is going to be costly for manufacturers; costs will undoubtedly be passed on to consumers. Inevitably many products will disappear—but the best will survive. This change is important. For instance, there is little or no health benefit for consumers buying fish oil supplements enriched in omega-3 fats if the product has become oxidized during manufacture or is contaminated with mercury. Similarly, we are only just beginning to appreciate the potential benefits of procyanidin products, and to define the optimal daily amount there will need to be large clinical trials of high-quality products.

Numerous clinical trials of vitamins and minerals have failed. In the 1970s and 1980s, consumption of beta-carotene was linked to lower levels of cancer, and experimental studies confirmed the benefit. Yet two major clinical trials studying the effects of beta-carotene supplements for smokers not only failed to show any benefit but actually found that the number of cancers and overall number of deaths increased in those receiving beta-carotene supplements. Surprisingly, this has not stopped the sale of beta-carotene supplements, which still are promoted as if they were a healthy alternative to eating vegetables.

The SU.VI.MAX (SUpplémentation en VItamines et Minéraux Antio-Xydants) Study in the Paris area is a more recent investigation of the benefits of a daily antioxidant vitamin combination (12 milligrams vitamin C, 30 milligrams vitamin E, 6 milligrams beta-carotene, 20 milligrams zinc, and 100 micrograms selenium) on more than 13,000 healthy people. After an average treatment period of seven and a half years, there was a trend for lower levels of cancer in men but no effect in women. The number of deaths was not altered by the treatment. The incidence of atherosclerosis appeared to increase in those receiving the supplement. This is evidence that there is no justification for taking these multipurpose supplements.

Various studies of vitamin E supplements have shown that taken in excess it can be harmful. An analysis of high-dose vitamin E studies was published in 2005. Daily doses of 150 IU (100 milligrams) or less had no harmful effects and sometimes were beneficial. Higher doses showed no benefit, and when the dose exceeded 400 IU (267 milligrams), adverse effects frequently were observed. It is hard to exceed 100 milligrams of vitamin E a day from dietary sources, so eating vitamin E–rich foods, such as avocados, nuts, and seeds, is the best way to ensure adequate intake.

High blood levels of homocysteine are associated with increased heart disease, particularly in people with diabetes. Homocysteine promotes oxidative stress and vascular inflammation, so its relationship to increased heart disease is not that surprising. Homocysteine levels increase because of various dietary and metabolic reasons, for example excessive meat consumption and inadequate intake of vegetables. The body cannot eliminate homocysteine without adequate folic acid. But the Norwegian Vitamin Trial (NORVIT) tested the efficacy of daily supplements of folic acid, vitamin B_6, and vitamin B_{12} on further cardiovascular events in 3,749 patients who had already had a heart attack. After three and a half years of follow-up, there was no evidence of any benefit. When this is compared with the results of the Italian trial mentioned on page 155, it is quite clear that complete dietary modification is essential and has greater success than any supplement treatment. This applies whether you are the victim of a heart attack or you are generally fit and healthy.

can SUPERFOODS save YOU?

Superfoods is a term used to describe foods with very high levels of naturally occurring vitamins or minerals. Broccoli, garlic, blueberries, and apples are just some of the many foods that have been hailed as superfoods over the past two decades.

Certainly, the vitamins and minerals we get from foods are more effective than those in supplements. Although we do not fully understand the processes involved, the many components of specific foods seem to work together in a way that manufactured supplements do not.

If we are to use food as therapy, however, the approach has to be a subtle one. If we were to eat portions of all the different superfoods that are recommended every day we may well end up exceeding the micronutrient intake needed for maximum benefit, or simply eating too much. We also might be excluding another important food.

remember

To satisfy all our dietary needs and promote optimal health, the best diets are composed of a wide range of nutritionally beneficial foods, which should be varied over a cycle of a week or more to keep the body supplied with all the essential vitamins and minerals. The important thing is to recognize the key foods you need to include in your diet on a regular basis—the goal of a healthy diet is complete nutrition.

11

a guide to complete nutrition

My DIET RECOMMENDATIONS are based on research (both mine and that of others) and observational studies to define the best eating patterns for providing all-round lifelong good health. The key principles are:

- Eat a good balance of healthy fats, carbohydrates, and proteins.
- Choose a variety of foods that contain plenty of vitamins and minerals.
- Harness the power of red wine and other polyphenol-rich foods and drinks to gain maximum protection for your blood vessels.

WHAT IS COMPLETE NUTRITION?

Most people are aware of the need for a balanced diet. Complete nutrition means eating foods that, together, contain the right balance of fats, carbohydrates, and proteins, and at the same time meet full vitamin and mineral requirements. For some people this may not differ much from the foods they eat already; it might be a simple matter of increasing the variety of foods. For others, certain eating habits lead to some foods being excluded from their diet; their choice of foods may be putting them at risk of deficiencies in a whole range of vitamins and minerals. This in turn increases their risk of cancer and heart disease and makes them more susceptible to many other illnesses because their immune systems are not properly equipped to fight infections. For instance, if you suffer from frequent colds, then the chances are your diet is deficient in one or more ways.

Carbohydrate, fat, and protein are known as macronutrients; they provide the body with energy, which is measured in calories (more accurately referred to as kilocalories) or kilojoules (kJ). Vitamins, minerals, and trace elements are called micronutrients; they do not provide any calories. Many people mainly eat calorie-rich foods that are lacking essential micronutrients. Such foods often contain a high level of refined carbohydrate and saturated fat. The concern is not just that these foods lead to obesity if eaten in excess (which they do), but also that they represent a nutritionally inadequate diet. Surveys of food consumption indicate that in many countries more than half the population has an inadequate intake of most vitamins and minerals. This is alarming because it puts these individuals at greater risk of many illnesses. Most vitamins and minerals are less well absorbed as the body ages, so there is an even greater need for older people to ensure adequate consumption, otherwise health can be rapidly compromised.

Health professionals now recognize poor diet as a major factor in many diseases. At the point of diagnosis many people realize that their bad habits have contributed to their ill health but think it is too late to change. It may not be possible to reverse all the damage, but many studies show that people who adopt good habits can improve their well-being and increase their life expectancy compared to people in a similar condition who are unwilling to modify their diet and/or lifestyle. So whatever your age, it is important to take matters into your own hands and start following a healthy diet—it's never too late! Regular exercise—even just walking upstairs—and eating more fruits and vegetables can increase your life expectancy over those in similar health who do not make these changes.

Your daily routine needs to form a pattern of activity and eating that provides sustainable good health—a complete nutrition lifestyle! The sooner you adopt this routine the more likely it is that it will become a lasting habit. It is important to identify which foods you lack in your diet and eat more of those, while reducing or avoiding foods that may be doing you harm or putting your health at risk. The latter particularly applies to processed foods containing high amounts of sugar, salt, or hydrogenated (trans) fats. This chapter highlights foods that can be used to boost the intake of specific vitamins and minerals while maintaining a balanced intake of carbohydrate, fat, and protein.

Information on the vitamin and mineral composition of foods can be found on the World's Healthiest Foods (www.whfoods.com) and Nutrition Data (www.nutrition-data.com) Web sites. The latter can help you find foods that are rich in specific nutrients and gives values based on your chosen portion size. It also has a recipe analysis function, which can show you how good or bad your current habits are and can help you adapt recipes to make them healthier. Detailed information on the role of vitamins and minerals in optimum nutrition can be found on the Web pages of the Linus Pauling Institute's Micronutrient Information Center (lpi.oregonstate.edu/infocenter).

GETTING THE BALANCE RIGHT

Recent diet research has shown that total daily calorie intake is best derived approximately 50 percent from carbohydrate, 30 percent from fat, and 20 percent from protein. For long-term good health, keeping to a daily meal plan that fits reasonably closely to this scheme is important. Of course, it is difficult to plan each meal to get the combination just right; the most important thing is mainly to eat healthy foods, and not overeat.

Thirty percent of calories from fat may sound like a lot: It represents 600 to 750 calories of the recommended daily average intake of 2000 to 2500 calories. But 600 to 750 calories would be provided by 5 to 6 tablespoons of olive oil, and many people eat far more fat than that! It's easy to forget just how much fat is hidden in snacks, cheese, cakes, and cookies.

The guideline daily intake of 2000 calories for women and 2500 for men is considerably more, or less, than many people need, as the chart below shows. Your age, body weight and shape, and activity level can make a big difference. Pregnant and breastfeeding women should consult their doctors.

To help you visualize the balance of nutrients on your plate, remember that fat has about 9 calories per gram, while protein and carbohydrate have about 4 calories per gram. Many foods contain a combination of protein, carbohydrate, and fat. The following example shows how you could achieve a healthy balance with a lunch of bean salad (add lemon juice, salt, and pepper):

RECOMMENDED DAILY CALORIE INTAKE

AGE	Very Sedentary			Moderately Active			Very Active		
	UNDER 30	30–60	OVER 60	UNDER 30	30–60	OVER 60	UNDER 30	30–60	OVER 60
Women									
126 lb/57 kg	1600	1570	1400	2000	1950	1750	2400	2350	2100
183 lb/83 kg	2050	1800	1700	2550	2270	2100	3070	2700	2500
Men									
140 lb/64 kg	1970	1900	1600	2470	2400	2000	2960	2870	2400
210 lb/95 kg	2540	2350	2040	3180	2940	2540	3100	3520	3050

	Carbohydrate (grams)	Fat (grams)	Protein (grams)
5.5 ounces canned red kidney beans	27	1	10
2 ounces green bell pepper	1.5	trace	0.5
1 tablespoon extra-virgin olive oil	0	12	0
3.5 ounces cottage cheese	3	4	12.5
1 apple	18	trace	0.5
TOTAL	49.5	17	23.5

A healthy pattern of eating can include all sorts of foods that most weight-loss diets tell you to avoid. For instance, a small amount of salami or chorizo sausage adds a delicious flavor to some recipes, and although it is high in fat it will not do any harm if eaten only occasionally. Many of the longest-lived people in Europe—in Sardinia and southwest France—regularly eat foods containing saturated fat. The important thing is that their diets are not primarily based on fatty foods. If you have very high cholesterol levels or need to lose weight, then you should restrict such foods, but if eaten occasionally they can increase the variety and taste of your meals.

DON'T FORGET YOUR GLASS OF WINE

Elsewhere in this book I have shown why I believe that daily consumption of red wine can improve your chances of living a longer, healthier life. The moderate amounts I recommend (no more than two 4-ounce glasses a day for women, three for men) would provide around 150 to 320 calories. You should take these calories into account in your daily total, particularly if you are trying to lose weight.

HUNGRY OR SATISFIED?

How do you eat enough to satisfy hunger without eating too much? Studies have shown that appetite is more readily satisfied by protein than fat, and by fat more than carbohydrate. So we should not be surprised that low-fat, high-carbohydrate diets result in people eating more than they need. What is the best way to achieve satiety? (Satiety is the feeling that you have eaten enough before you have eaten too much, and which leaves you without any sense of hunger or desire to eat until the next meal.)

When a carbohydrate-rich meal is digested, sugars are absorbed into the bloodstream, which stimulates insulin secretion from the pancreas. This is a normal physiological response—fat and muscle tissues depend on insulin to trigger the uptake of sugar from the blood. If carbohydrate is digested too quickly, the sugar levels in the blood rise so rapidly that an excess of insulin is produced, which increases appetite further. So refined starchy and sugary carbohydrates tend to drive people to eat more than they should. This underlies the science advising you to choose carbohydrates that are less readily digestible; they are described as having a lower glycemic (glucose, or blood sugar) index, or GI. Foods also need to contain fewer total calories from digestible carbohydrates; the available sugar from a food after digestion is referred to as the glycemic load, or GL.

It is a good general principle mainly to eat foods with a low GI and low GL and avoid high-GL sugary foods and refined grain products such as white bread and white rice. Most vegetables and pulses and many fresh fruits (including berries, citrus fruits, apples, pears, cherries, peaches, and plums) have a low GL. Minimally processed whole-grain products such as oats, barley, whole-wheat bread, and bread made with seeds and nuts have medium to low GI and GL—the carbohydrates they contain are digested slowly and create only a small rise in insulin production.

Another factor influencing appetite is the bulk of food—if your stomach is full your appetite decreases. Vegetables and salads provide bulk because they are high in dietary fiber. So eating plenty of vegetables will make you less hungry—and vegetables also provide a wide range of valuable vitamins and minerals.

When a fatty or protein-rich meal is digested, it stimulates the release of a variety of gut hormones into the blood. These hormones send signals to the brain to stop you from eating more. Also, when protein is digested, it is broken down into amino acids. There is no mechanism for storing specific amino acids in the body, so once the daily needs for protein synthesis are met, the excess is metabolized by the body to produce energy. This occurs relatively slowly, so amino acids from protein foods provide a slow-release form of energy, which can stop you from feeling hungry.

WHAT'S SO GOOD ABOUT a mediterranean diet?

Research has shown that a Mediterranean-style diet can improve heart health. Recommendations are based on the Cretan diet of the 1960s and 1970s. This gives a good balance of fat, carbohydrate, and protein, with ample fruits and vegetables.

The Cretan diet of thirty to forty years ago had many features that we now recognize as healthy habits: regular meals of fish, plenty of vegetables, whole-grain foods, pulses (beans, chickpeas, and lentils), seeds, and nuts. The small amount of meat came from animals and birds that grazed on local grasses and plants rather than being fed on grains. This meant that the meat, cheese, yogurt, milk, and eggs were naturally high in omega-3 polyunsaturated fats. The overall diet provided a roughly equal intake of omega-3 and omega-6 polyunsaturated fats, which is considered the ideal ratio. Because the main sources of protein are fish, pulses, and vegetables, consumption of saturated fat is reduced. Clinical studies have shown repeatedly that this type of diet is best for lowering blood pressure, improving cholesterol levels, and increasing longevity by reducing the risk of heart disease and cancer.

Some people are surprised to learn that the Cretan diet was relatively high in fat (up to 35 percent of energy from fat). However, the main fat used was olive oil, which consists of approximately 70 percent monounsaturated fat, with low amounts of saturated and polyunsaturated fat.

Another key aspect of the Mediterranean diet is the emphasis on eating plenty of fresh fruits and vegetables. The risk of having a stroke is 20 to 30 percent lower for people who eat more than five servings of fruits and vegetables a day. This can be attributed partly to the blood pressure-lowering effect of higher potassium consumption. Equally importantly, eating large amounts of fruits and vegetables increases the intake of a wide range of vitamins, minerals, and other plant chemicals, which have additional protective properties. Variety is important, as different vegetables and fruits are rich in different nutrients. Even so-called superfoods—apples, blueberries, cabbage, or anything else—should not be eaten in excess, to the exclusion of others.

If bananas and potatoes are the only fruits and vegetables you eat, you will not be getting the variety of vitamins and minerals you need. In addition, potatoes and bananas generally have a medium GL; if the glycemic load of the food you eat is too high, your appetite will not be satisfied for long. If you are trying to lose weight, then overall consumption of potatoes and bananas should be reduced, but I don't think they need be avoided altogether. Interestingly, new potatoes have a lower GL than other potatoes.

FIVE A DAY—AT LEAST!

Recommendations vary from five, to nine, to as many as twelve servings of fruits and vegetables a day. A serving is defined as about 80 grams. Another way to think about this is as 1⅔ to 2¼ pounds for a man (nine to twelve portions) and as 1⅛ to 1⅔ pounds for a woman. When I first read this, I thought it sounded like gluttony, but when I weighed a selection of fruits and vegetables

If you feel you need to change your eating habits, what is the best strategy? American nutritionist Dr. Ancel Keys was the first to highlight the benefits of a Cretan-style Mediterranean diet, and he lived to be 100. So why not start by following his example? Eat more beans, lentils, chickpeas, and nuts instead of red meat, and eat plenty of vegetables and fruits. The Mediterranean diet is also high in monounsaturated fat (mainly from olive oil), high in complex carbohydrates (from vegetables, fruits, and minimally processed grains) and uses virtually no added sugar; it has an excellent mix of nutrients for providing general good health. Substantial research supports the benefits of this way of eating, as discussed in previous chapters.

that I could imagine eating each day, I realized that this would be a reasonable amount if it were served over the whole day, at breakfast, lunch, and dinner.

Some nutritionists do not count potatoes as a serving of vegetables. I think it is fine to include a portion of boiled or microwaved new potatoes in their skins two or three times a week. Potatoes are a surprisingly good source of vitamin C, and when eaten with their skins they can add valuable trace elements. But don't start counting french fries as a side salad!

"GREEK" SALAD?

Since November 2004, the U.S. Food and Drug Administration has allowed a qualified health claim on the labeling of olive oil: "Limited and not conclusive scientific evidence suggests that eating about 2 tablespoons of olive oil per day may reduce the risk of coronary heart disease." Of course, this is not in addition to what you already eat: it is meant to replace saturated fats in your diet, so you need to stop eating other fatty foods. I wish the olive oil message had gotten through at street level. At the salad bars of some restaurants it is not uncommon to find that when you order a Greek salad the only dressing offered is low fat. No olive oil can be found on the premises.

FRUIT AND VEGETABLES—PICK YOUR OWN

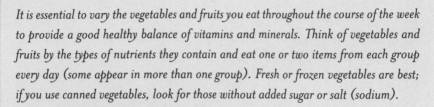

It is essential to vary the vegetables and fruits you eat throughout the course of the week to provide a good healthy balance of vitamins and minerals. Think of vegetables and fruits by the types of nutrients they contain and eat one or two items from each group every day (some appear in more than one group). Fresh or frozen vegetables are best; if you use canned vegetables, look for those without added sugar or salt (sodium).

RICH IN VITAMIN C

Fruits: blackberries, black currants, blueberries, clementines, cranberries, grapefruit, guava, kiwis, lemons, limes, lychees, mandarins, oranges, papaya, pineapple, raspberries, red currants, strawberries, tangerines

Vegetables: broccoli, Brussels sprouts, kale, potatoes, red cabbage, romaine lettuce, bell peppers, spinach, tomatoes, watercress, zucchini,

RICH IN FOLIC ACID

Vegetables: arugula, asparagus, avocados, beans and peas (dried), broccoli, cauliflower, globe artichokes, green cabbage, spinach, watercress

Fruit: oranges

RICH IN CAROTENOIDS

Vegetables: broccoli, butternut squash, carrots, corn, green beans, green and red bell peppers, kale, pumpkin, radicchio, spinach, sweet potatoes, tomatoes, watercress

Fruits: apricots, mangoes, melon (orange–fleshed), papaya, passion fruit

RICH IN POLYPHENOLS

Fruits: apples, blackberries, black currants, blueberries, cranberries, kaki fruit, persimmons, pomegranates, raspberries, red currants, strawberries

RICH IN MINERALS OR OTHER MICRONUTRIENTS

Vegetables: beans (dried), chickpeas, lentils, tofu

RICH IN CARBOHYDRATES

Vegetables: beans (dried), beets, broad beans, celeriac, corn, chickpeas, green peas, Jerusalem artichokes, lentils, parsnips, potatoes, tofu

RICH IN PRE-BIOTICS

Vegetables: asparagus, endive/chicory, Jerusalem artichokes, leeks, onions

OTHER VEGETABLES

celery, cucumber, eggplant, green cabbage, lettuce, mushrooms, okra, radishes, scallions

OTHER FRUITS

cherries, dates, figs, grapes, nectarines, peaches, pears, plums

PROTEIN—HOW MUCH AND WHAT IS BEST?

The optimum protein intake is about 20 percent of total calories, with 50 percent of calories coming from carbohydrates. Many diets still recommend around 15 percent protein. But an eating pattern that includes slightly more protein is more satisfying and may help you control your appetite better. Some dietary guidelines recommend a slightly higher protein intake (20 to 30 percent) to help lose weight and to provide a metabolic balance, particularly in individuals with diabetes or who are overweight with a sedentary lifestyle and at risk of developing type 2 diabetes. Higher protein intakes for short periods probably do little harm, but generally I think it is better to maintain protein at around 20 percent of calorie intake. This will help you to avoid the kidney problems or gout that can be triggered by high-protein diets. Some popular diets focus on high protein intake from meat, poultry, fish, and dairy foods. While they can help you lose weight in the short term, they are far from ideal for lifelong good health (see pages 142 to 144).

Many other foods contain a proportion of protein, in combination with fats and carbohydrates. Pulses, grains, nuts, and seeds are good sources of protein, and there's a small amount of protein in many vegetables. In a number of clinical studies, an increased intake of protein from vegetable sources has been shown to have health benefits, particularly lower blood pressure, which in turn reduces the risk of heart disease.

Beans, lentils, dried peas, and chickpeas (collectively known as pulses or legumes) typically have about two and a half times more carbohydrate than

COUNT YOUR CHICKENS

Many diets suggest that because chicken and turkey are low in fat, they are therefore healthier choices than red meat. However, the way poultry is reared in the modern world often results in poor-quality meat that is higher in saturated fat and also has a higher ratio of omega-6 to omega-3 fats than the poultry of thirty or forty years ago.

Although organic chicken is a better choice than standard chicken, it is still hard to know what the quality of the animal's diet is likely to have been in terms of omega-3 fats. Nowadays even organic producers are under pressure to produce as intensively as they can within the organic guidelines.

Small portions of meat such as lamb or beef can be as healthy as chicken if the meat is lean and of the very best quality. This means the animal needs to have grown naturally, grazing in fields or on hills. Look for meat that has been grass fed, as it will have more omega-3 polyunsaturated fatty acids. In the case of pork, as with chicken, it is impossible to know what the animal has been reared on even with an organic diet.

Instead of having corn-fed chicken every other day, believing that it is the healthiest option, why not have small portions of high-quality meat or poultry two or three times a week and eat fish, nuts, beans, or lentils on other days? Such variety is a better choice for health.

protein—ideal if you want to obtain 50 percent of your calories from carbohydrate and 20 percent from protein.

Most pulses are low in fat. Soybeans are an exception, in that they contain approximately 20 percent fat, although this is a fairly healthy mix of roughly 15 to 20 percent saturated fat, 20 to 25 percent monounsaturated fat, and 7 to 8 percent omega-3 and 50 percent omega-6 polyunsaturated fats. Soybeans also contain a higher ratio of protein to carbohydrate than other beans. This all adds up to a very nutritious option and explains why soy protein is considered one of the best substitutes for meat. Soybeans and tofu (soybean curd) have little flavor and are best combined with other, tastier, ingredients. Soy flour adds protein to breads and baked items. The downside is confusion over the potential risks of genetically modified (GM) beans. There is some concern that GM soy is linked to increased occurrence of soy allergies. This will need to be monitored carefully, as it may be one of the strongest arguments for eating only organically grown GM-free beans.

To obtain 20 percent of your calorie intake from protein means 400 to 500 calories of a daily intake of 2000 to 2500 calories. The following sources of protein are generally low in fat and will help you plan your meals. Serve them with healthy carbohydrate-rich foods such as brown rice or whole-wheat pasta, and plenty of vegetables.

FOOD	SERVING SIZE	CALORIES FROM PROTEIN	TOTAL CALORIES PER SERVING
White fish, baked	6.5 ounces	168	193
Salmon fillet, broiled	5 ounces	142	258
Shrimp, boiled	2 ounces	50	57
Chicken breast, skinless, broiled	4 ounces	146	168
Lamb chop, grilled, fat cut off	3 ounces	99	181
Lean beef steak, broiled	5 ounces	176	250
Egg, boiled	1 large egg (1¾ ounces)	24	75
Chickpeas, canned	3.5 ounces	27	109
Lentils, green, boiled	4 ounces	40	123
Tofu, steamed	3 ounces	27	62
Cottage cheese	4 ounces	56	116

Proteins are composed of twenty different amino acids. Eight of these are referred to as essential amino acids (isoleucine, leucine, lysine, methionine, phenylalanine, threonine, tryptophan, and valine) because we rely on dietary sources to stay healthy. Infants also need histidine and arginine. Some vegetable proteins have lower levels of one or more essential amino acids, so while it is a good idea to increase your consumption of vegetable proteins, it is important that you choose a variety of different pulses, nuts, seeds, grains, and vegetables throughout the day and over the course of a week. This will ensure that you are not missing out on any essential amino acids.

Eating foods rich in the amino acid arginine can boost blood vessel function. This is because arginine helps ensure optimal production of nitric oxide, which acts as a vasodilator and helps prevent blood clots from forming. This does not mean I am recommending arginine supplements. A clinical trial of arginine supplementation in patients who recently had had a heart attack found that it could be harmful. Adequate arginine intake can be achieved through normal consumption of either vegetable or animal protein foods.

Two tablespoons (about 1 ounce) of pumpkin seeds provides more than 1 gram of arginine; other seeds, pulses, and nuts are also good sources of arginine.

GOOD CARBS, BAD CARBS

When it comes to carbohydrates, the best choice is undoubtedly whole-grain foods, such as whole-grain breakfast cereals, unprocessed oats, whole-wheat bread and pasta, and brown rice. These are also sources of protein, vitamins, and minerals. Analysis of weight gain in the Health Professionals Follow-up Study has shown that the lowest weight gain was in those subjects eating whole-grain foods as part of a healthy pattern of eating.

Unfortunately, far too many people in industrialized societies eat too many refined and processed grain products, such as white bread and white rice. Cakes, cookies, and other sweetened baked products are foods to be avoided. These are generally calorie-rich, nutrient-poor food choices. Commercial products are also often high in trans fats (see pages 140 to 141). Nibbling cookies while you work is one of the worst habits you can have if you want to lose weight and stay healthy. Pizza, particularly the thick-crust variety, is another bad choice: high GI, high GL, high in salt, and often, depending on the topping, high in saturated fats. Pizza is also generally a very poor source of vitamins. I'm not saying you can never have a slice of pizza again, but it should be an occasional part of a well-balanced diet, and it should always be accompanied by plenty of vegetables or salad.

A BALANCED INTAKE OF FATS

I recommend that 30 percent of total calories should come from fat. Based on the Mediterranean diet, approximately two-thirds of calories from fat should be from monounsaturated fat (such as olive oil, nuts, and avocados), and the remaining third should be half from polyunsaturated fatty acids (PUFAs) and half from saturated fat. PUFAs should not make up more than a third of your fat intake (i.e., 10 percent of total calorie intake). On food labels look for foods with a saturated fat content that is less than one-fifth of the total amount of fat.

Both omega-3 and omega-6 PUFAs play an important role in maintaining optimal health. Because they can be obtained only through dietary sources, they are referred to as essential fatty acids. DHA (docosahexaenoic acid, the most important type of omega-3 PUFA) is particularly important in the brain. Low levels have been linked to increased likelihood of dementia in the elderly and higher prevalence of Attention Deficit Disorder (ADD) in children and young adults. Adequate consumption during pregnancy is essential to allow the baby's brain to develop healthily.

Many food sources of PUFAs contain a mix of omega-3 and omega-6 fatty acids. However, some popular vegetable oils, such as corn, sunflower, and safflower, have very high amounts of omega-6 and no omega-3 PUFAs. These oils are widely used in the food industry, and the typical diet in industrialized countries forces overconsumption of omega-6 PUFAs. Excessive consumption of omega-6 fatty acids with inadequate consumption of omega-3 fatty acids has been linked to an increased risk of heart disease, asthma, and allergies, as well as various inflammatory conditions such as arthritis and inflammatory bowel disease. If you want to improve your PUFA balance, you should avoid these oils as much as possible.

To achieve the ideal 1 to 1 ratio of omega-3 to omega-6 PUFA it is important to balance foods containing omega-6 PUFAs with foods that are rich in omega-3 PUFAs such as oily fish and flaxseed. Flaxseed is the best plant source of omega-3 PUFAs, with approximately three to four times more omega-3 than omega-6. The type of omega-3 PUFA from plant sources, alpha-linolenic acid, is converted in your body to eicosapentaenoic acid (EPA), and then to DHA. However, this occurs inefficiently, and perhaps not at all if omega-6 PUFA consumption greatly exceeds that of omega-3.

Canola oil and hemp seeds are rich in alpha-linolenic acid (an omega-3 PUFA), but this still only represents 25 to 30 percent of the amount of linoleic acid (omega-6 PUFA).

PUFAs are easily damaged by excessive heat, both during manufacture and when used for cooking. Always look for the better-quality, cold-pressed (virgin) oils, which are available in health food stores. Cooking at high temperatures destroys alpha-linolenic acid, so canola oil is unsuitable for frying. Olive oil is a good choice because it contains a high proportion of monounsaturated fat, which means that the omega-6 to omega-3 ratio is less significant. Flaxseed oil is too unstable for use in cooking; it should be kept in the fridge and used to make a nutty-tasting dressing for salads and vegetables. Ground flaxseed can be sprinkled over savory dishes, on yogurt with fruit, or mixed with muesli for breakfast.

Oily fish is the best source of omega-3, in the form of DHA. But in the near future it is unlikely to be environmentally sustainable for us all to meet our needs through this route. Relying on fish and seafood for omega-3 PUFAs also raises concerns because of the likelihood of contamination by mercury, cadmium, and other pollutants. Availability of uncontaminated fish is likely to get worse rather than better. Farmed fish may not be the answer unless farming is carefully regulated. The diet of farmed fish may be supplemented with foods containing excessive omega-6 PUFAs, so the product reaching the consumer is no longer the best choice to meet DHA needs. Alternative strategies are called for.

If you want to rely on your body to make your own DHA, flaxseed is a good starting point in a diet where omega-3 and omega-6 PUFAs are kept to approximately equal amounts. However, flaxseed can have a laxative action in some people. Walnuts are another good source of omega-3 PUFAs. Green vegetables such as broccoli, kale, spinach, and watercress do not have high levels of fat but the small amounts present are mainly omega-3 PUFAs. Yet another good reason to eat your greens!

Choosing meat from grass-fed animals can help, because they have already converted some of the alpha-linolenic acid into EPA and DHA. Production of omega-3 enriched eggs has become quite common. Sometimes this is achieved by feeding the chickens flaxseed-based foods; in other cases fishmeal is used. The latest innovation in this area is to grow carefully selected phytoplankton in fermenters; these microscopic plants synthesize DHA, which can be extracted and used to supplement foods for human or animal consumption. Various approaches to substituting for oily fish in the diet are likely to become more common over the next few years. In the process it is likely that the ideal daily intake of DHA will be defined.

eat more nuts

Nuts mainly contain healthy monounsaturated and polyunsaturated fats. Clinical studies of diets that include daily nut consumption show a decrease in LDL-cholesterol (the bad form of cholesterol) of up to 10 percent. Nuts are also good sources of protein, vitamins, and minerals, and can make a valuable contribution to a healthy diet. Nuts contain B vitamins (B_1, B_2, and B_3), vitamin E (particularly almonds and hazelnuts), copper, iron, manganese, magnesium, phosphorus, and zinc.

In the past, diet advice usually included avoiding nuts because they were considered fattening. Yes, they are calorie rich. Eating large amounts of nuts without cutting back on other foods will not help you lose weight. However, nuts added to salads or included in baked savory dishes can act as a substitute for meat. As a snack, nuts will satisfy your appetite because they contain protein and fat. Nutritionally they are a good combination with cereals, which makes muesli (see recipe, page 224) a good start to the day. If you choose peanuts or other nuts in their shells, the process of shelling them can slow you down and may stop you from eating too many. Salted nuts do not count as a healthy snack. But a few chocolate-covered nuts, if the chocolate coating is 70 percent cocoa solids and contains no vegetable oil trans fats, can be a healthy choice, in moderation.

If you are allergic to nuts, you need to eat other foods rich in monounsaturated fat, vegetable protein, vitamin E, and other micronutrients. Pulses and seeds are sources of vegetable protein. Avocados are rich in monounsaturated fat, vitamin E, and folate.

fat-soluble vitamins, and where to find them

VITAMIN A is important for healthy skin and hair, good eyesight, and reproductive function in both sexes. Dry, scaly skin and poor night vision are early signs of vitamin A deficiency. Virtually every cell of the body needs vitamin A. Many of its effects are subtle changes in cell function that allow cells to thrive and the body to fight off infection. Frequent viral infections may be the result of inadequate vitamin A intake.

The term *vitamin A* describes a range of similar natural chemicals known as retinoids. Preformed vitamin A is found in high amounts in liver; butter and cheese are other sources. However, it is not necessary to eat animal products to have adequate amounts because the body can also make vitamin A from carotenoids (the yellow, orange, and red pigments in many vegetables and fruits) such as beta-carotene. Carrots, parsley, green vegetables, squash, sweet potatoes, orange-fleshed melons, tomatoes, bell peppers, and papayas are rich sources of carotenoids. With green vegetables it is not always obvious that they are a source of carotenoids because the green of chlorophyll masks the orange-yellow color. Some carotenoids have specific roles: Lutein and zeaxanthin, for instance, are essential for a healthy retina and can reduce the risk of sight loss from age-related macular degeneration. Kale, Swiss chard, spinach, watercress, and other leafy dark green vegetables—and radicchio—are good sources of lutein and other carotenoids.

FOOD	SERVING SIZE	VITAMIN A EQUIVALENT (MCG)/(IU)
Chicken liver, sautéed	2 ounces	2400 (8000)
Carrot, boiled	1 medium (2 ounces)	3000 (9600)
Spinach, boiled	3 ounces	2641 (8800)
Sweet potato, baked	6 ounces	6570 (21900)
Kale, boiled	3 ounces	3400 (11333)

Some leafy greens should be eaten every day to provide adequate carotenoids to meet daily vitamin A requirements.

Daily intake of vitamin A should be 600 micrograms for women and 700 micrograms for men; vitamin A equivalent from carotenoids can never reach unsafe levels, because the body converts only what it needs. However, 3000 micrograms of preformed vitamin A from dietary sources is considered a safe maximum limit. Vitamin A supplements are not recommended because consumption in excess of 1500 micrograms per day has been linked to an increased risk of bone fractures and osteoporosis. Excess intake in pregnant women (greater than 7500 micrograms a day) can cause fetal malformation. To avoid excess intake of vitamin A during pregnancy, it is generally recommended that pregnant women avoid eating liver.

VITAMIN D helps your body to absorb calcium and phosphorus, to make healthy bones and teeth. It is therefore important for preventing osteoporosis,

---

VITAMINS AND MINERALS

When you see recommended intakes for vitamins and minerals, you may be confused by the various terms used: RDA (Recommended Dietary Allowance), DRI (Dietary Reference Index), DV (Daily Value), AI (Adequate Intake), and EAR (Estimated Average Requirement). Sometimes values have not been fully assessed: You may see the term ESAD-DI (estimated safe and adequate daily dietary intake). Some recommendations are for the minimum intake needed to prevent nutritional deficiencies in the majority of the population. Individuals vary in their nutritional needs throughout life; stress, illness, and smoking increase the body's need for nutrients. Some daily intakes are calculated for a person of average weight—if you are overweight, you may need slightly more. Some nutritionists recommend higher intakes because they believe these can be beneficial for optimum nutrition.

The daily intakes I recommend should benefit most adults; many are based on the WHO/FAO report Human Vitamin and Mineral Requirements.

If you are pregnant or breastfeeding, you will need higher intakes of most micronutrients, but you should be especially careful not to exceed recommended intakes of others. Consult your doctor for individual advice.

and it also improves immune function. Adequate vitamin D also reduces the risk of various types of cancer, while lack of this vitamin has been linked to autoimmune diseases such as multiple sclerosis and rheumatoid arthritis.

Vitamin D can be made in the skin on exposure to sunlight; fifteen minutes a day should be enough for most people.

Oily fish is the best food source of vitamin D, and supplements such as cod liver oil capsules are a popular alternative. Shrimp, egg yolks, and milk are other sources. Breakfast cereals, margarine, and reduced-fat spreads are often fortified with vitamin D. If you eat a lot of these foods, I do not recommend that you take a supplement, as you might then consume too much.

Daily intake should be 5 to 10 micrograms a day; 15 micrograms for those over sixty-six years old; exceeding 50 micrograms can be harmful. During winter months, or if you never expose your skin to sunlight, you will need to obtain vitamin D from food or supplements.

VITAMIN E is an important antioxidant vitamin. It helps prevent oxidation of cell membranes, which keeps them flexible and therefore protects the health of all cells, including skin, blood, nerves, and muscles. It strengthens the immune system and may reduce the risk of heart disease by preventing oxidation of LDL-cholesterol.

Vitamin E works most effectively when there is also adequate vitamin C consumption. Vitamin E deficiency is uncommon. However, low-fat diets decrease the intake of foods containing vitamin E, and also reduce the body's ability to absorb it. Sunflower seeds, hazelnuts, and almonds are rich sources of vitamin E. Pine nuts, Brazil and other nuts, peanut butter, and avocados can also make significant contributions to vitamin E intake. Other

FOOD	SERVING SIZE	VITAMIN D (MCG)/(IU)
Mackerel, broiled	6 ounces	15 (600)
Salmon, canned	2 ounces	5 (200)
Sardines, canned	2 ounces	3 (120)
Milk, low-fat (1.8 percent fat)	8 ounces	2.5 (100)
Egg, poached	1 large	1 (40)

foods that contain some vitamin E include blackberries, mangoes, tomatoes, chickpeas, broccoli, asparagus, watercress, and spinach.

Daily intake for adults should be 10 milligrams. Studies of supplement takers show that exceeding 100 milligrams a day confers no greater benefit and may even be linked to increased risk of coronary events.

FOOD	SERVING SIZE	VITAMIN E (MG)/(IU)
Avocado	½ pear (2.5 ounces)	1.5 (2.25)
Hazelnuts	10 nuts	2 (3)
Sunflower seeds	1 tablespoon	5.5 (8.25)
Blackberries	3 ounces	2 (3)
Mango	1 (5 ounces)	1.5 (2.25)

VITAMIN K is a vitamin that is rarely talked about. It is essential for normal blood clotting and bone formation, and helps prevent osteoporosis. Babies receive an injection of vitamin K at birth, but that is usually the only time deficiency is likely. It is abundant in green vegetables and herbs (such as parsley, basil, Swiss chard, spinach, lettuce (most types, but not iceberg), cabbage, broccoli, asparagus, Brussels sprouts, scallions, and seaweed). Soybeans and other pulses, fruits (prunes, kiwi, blackberries), eggs, nuts, and whole-grain foods can also supply useful amounts. The gut bacteria make vitamin K, but it is not clear whether this makes any contribution to daily requirements.

Daily intake for an adult should be 55 micrograms for women and 65 micrograms for men.

WATER-SOLUBLE VITAMINS, AND WHERE TO FIND THEM

B-group vitamins have many metabolic functions. They enable cells to grow, generate energy from food, and synthesize proteins. Although some B vitamins have specific roles, such as producing red blood cells, collectively they work in synergy to maintain a healthy nervous system, digestive system,

FOOD	SERVING SIZE	VITAMIN K (MCG)
Prunes	6	36
Parsley	1 tablespoon	61
Brussels sprouts	3 ounces	120
Lettuce or arugula	2 ounces	57
Kiwi	1 medium (3 ounces)	34

liver, muscles, brain, hair, eyes, and skin. Deficiency in one or more B vitamins can cause fatigue, forgetfulness, inflammation of skin and mucous membranes, anemia, muscle and heart problems, and nervous system disorders. This group includes B_1 (thiamin), B_2 (riboflavin), B_3 (niacin), B_5 (pantothenic acid), B_6 (pyridoxine), B_{12} (cyanocobalamin), and folate (folic acid). B_3 is the only B vitamin that is stable during cooking—the others may be degraded partially or completely depending on the type of food and cooking time. A healthy, varied diet should supply adequate amounts of most B vitamins.

B_1 (THIAMIN) is present in the husk (bran) of whole grains, so whole-wheat bread, whole-wheat pasta, brown rice, and rolled oats are good sources. Sunflower seeds, peanuts, and various other seeds and nuts have reasonable amounts, and it's also found in egg yolks, fish, and pulses.

B FORTIFIED

In many countries, the refined flour used for bread and other baked products is fortified with certain B vitamins, as well as calcium and iron. In the United States, Canada, Chile, and other countries, refined flour is also fortified with folic acid; this is still under discussion in Europe. Many breakfast cereals are also fortified. Basically this is because manufacturers are required to replace the vitamins that are lost during processing. If you are looking for easy options, you can meet most of your vitamin B requirements from these products. The problem is that these foods tend to have a high GI value (in other words, they contain easily digestible carbohydrate that stimulates excessive insulin production); this makes such products a poor food choice.

FOOD	SERVING SIZE	THIAMIN (MG)
Sunflower seeds	1 tablespoon (0.5 ounces)	0.4
Whole-wheat bread	2 slices (2.5 ounces)	0.2
Whole-wheat pasta, boiled	5 ounces	0.3
Pork, lean loin chop, broiled	1 chop, excluding bone (3 ounces)	1
Soybeans, green, boiled	3 ounces	0.3

Pork, bacon, and ham are good sources of thiamin. Daily intake should be 1.1 milligrams for women and 1.2 milligrams for men.

B₂ (RIBOFLAVIN) is found in the greatest amounts in almonds, cheese, and other dairy products, eggs, mackerel, herring, sardines, soy flour, liver, venison, beef, lamb, and duck. Daily intake should be 1.1 milligrams for women and 1.3 milligrams for men.

FOOD	SERVING SIZE	RIBOFLAVIN (MG)
Almonds	1 ounce	0.2
Camembert cheese	1 ounce	0.2
Yogurt	4 ounces	0.2
Venisona steak, broiled	3.5 ounces	0.6
Mackerel, broiled	5 ounces	0.5

B₃ (NIACIN) can be obtained from fish, chicken, turkey, lean meat, mushrooms, grains, nuts, and seeds. Daily intake should be 14 milligrams for women and 16 milligrams for men.

FOOD	SERVING SIZE	NIACIN (MG)
Mushrooms, stir-fried	3 ounces	2.7
Tuna, canned in water	3 ounces	11
Turkey breast, roasted	1 ounce	6
Peanut butter	3 ounces	4
Beef, lean steak, broiled	5 ounces	8

VITAMIN B₅ (PANTOTHENIC ACID) is found in a wide variety of foods. Nuts, seeds, and avocados are good sources, but most foods contain some

B_5, so an adequate intake is easily achieved with a varied healthy diet. Daily intake should be 5 milligrams for most adults.

VITAMIN B_6 (PYRIDOXINE) is also a fairly common. Nuts, fish, poultry, and lean meat are good sources, as are bananas and avocados. Daily intake should be 1.3 milligrams for most adults, rising to 1.5 milligrams for women over fifty and 1.7 milligrams for men over fifty.

VITAMIN B_{12} is present in small amounts in all foods of animal origin, including fish and shellfish, lean meat and poultry, eggs, milk, yogurt, and cheese. Deficiency is generally considered unlikely unless you are a strict vegetarian or vegan or you have problems with absorption from the intestines; vegans should take a supplement. However, many people do not have an optimum intake and there is increasing evidence linking vitamin B_{12} deficiency to dementia (see following page).

Liver is a rich source of B_2, B_3, B_5, B_6, B_{12}, and folic acid: a 2-ounce portion can more than meet daily needs for B_2 and B_{12}. In fact, it contains more than a week's supply of vitamin B_{12}. Unlike most water-soluble vitamins, vitamin B_{12} is stored in the human liver, so a serving of liver once every two weeks will provide all the vitamin B_{12} you need. Many diets recommend avoiding liver because of high amounts of saturated fat and cholesterol; I think this advice is flawed. A 2-ounce portion of calf's, lamb's, or chicken liver contains less than 2 grams of saturated fat, and cholesterol from the food you eat is poorly absorbed, so the effect on your blood cholesterol levels will be insignificant. Daily intake for most adults should be 2.4 micrograms a day.

FOLATE is the naturally occurring form of this vitamin, folic acid is the synthetic form found in supplements and added to fortified foods. It is an important synergist for the actions of B vitamins, particularly B_6 and B_{12}. Although folate deficiency has to be severe before symptoms such as anemia occur, low consumption of folate is a health risk because it increases the risk of heart disease and cancer.

Excess alcohol consumption interferes with the absorption of many B vitamins and folate. Long-term overconsumption of alcohol may be recognized by the symptoms of B vitamin deficiency. For women who regularly

VITAMIN B$_{12}$ FOR A HEALTHY BRAIN

The absorption of vitamin B$_{12}$ is more complex than it is for most vitamins. When a meal is eaten, the stomach wall produces acid and a digestive enzyme called pepsin. These act together to break down proteins and release vitamin B$_{12}$ from food. The body also produces a key protein called intrinsic factor, which binds the vitamin B$_{12}$ to protect it during transit through the intestines until it is absorbed.

Approximately 10 to 15 percent of people over sixty-five are vitamin B$_{12}$ deficient. Most doctors consider poor vitamin B$_{12}$ status as a likely cause of anemia, but it also increases the risk of heart disease and the likelihood of depression, reduces cognitive performance, and hastens the development and progression of dementia.

There are two main reasons for poor absorption of vitamin B$_{12}$ in the elderly: insufficient acid production in the stomach and lack of intrinsic factor. Gastric atrophy, a lack of function in the stomach wall, may underlie both the lack of acid production and the reduction in intrinsic factor. Why is gastric atrophy such a problem in the elderly? The main factor is infection by Helicobacter pylori. *The infection may be present in the stomach for many years without causing any major symptoms, but eventually it leads to loss of healthy function. The good news is that red wine drinkers are reported to have some resistance to* Helicobacter pylori *infection.*

There are several other causes of poor vitamin B$_{12}$ absorption. Pernicious anemia is present in 1 to 2 percent of people over sixty-five. This is an autoimmune condition in which antibodies have developed to intrinsic factor and so prevent it from functioning. Another potentially common cause is excessive use of medications that interfere with the stomach's acid production; other medications can also affect vitamin B$_{12}$ absorption. Because poor vitamin B$_{12}$ status is fairly common in the elderly, supplements should be considered.

drink moderate amounts of alcohol, eating foods rich in folate appears to reduce the risk of breast cancer. Similarly, increased folate intake helps reduce the risk of colon cancer in all alcohol drinkers.

Folate is essential for the healthy development of babies; pregnant women and women who might become pregnant should make sure they consume adequate amounts. In order to prevent neural tube defects, a folic acid supplement (400 micrograms a day) should be taken before conception and until week twelve of pregnancy.

Green vegetables (especially asparagus, broccoli, Brussels sprouts, spinach, and kale), cauliflower, soy flour, many varieties of beans, and liver are good sources of folic acid. Fruits, avocados, sunflower seeds, nuts, and cheese are moderate sources. Daily intake for most adults should be 200 to 400 micrograms a day.

FOOD	SERVING SIZE	FOLATE (MCG)
Asparagus, boiled	6 spears (5 ounces)	225
Broccoli, boiled	3 ounces	75
Spinach, boiled	3 ounces	95
Orange	1 medium (5 ounces)	45
Hazelnuts	1 ounce	28

BIOTIN is another water-soluble vitamin that is generally grouped with B vitamins, as it synergizes with them. It is essential for fat metabolism as well as for the production of energy from other sources. Because biotin is found in many foods, deficiency does not often occur. The intestinal flora also synthesize biotin. However, raw egg whites contain a protein called avidin that binds biotin irreversibly, so eating uncooked egg whites, for example in mousses and other desserts, can prevent its absorption.

VITAMIN C (ASCORBIC ACID) is the classic vitamin that everybody knows comes from citrus fruits and is essential to avoid scurvy—the scourge of sailors of old. Vitamin C is a potent antioxidant and increases the effectiveness of vitamin E. Vitamin C acts as an antioxidant in the aqueous environment of cells, while vitamin E does the same job in the lipid or fatty cellular components. Vitamin C needs to be eaten every day; it cannot be stored in the body and any excess is filtered through the kidneys.

Vitamin C is best obtained from fresh fruits and vegetables. The amounts in foods decrease with storage. Oranges and freshly squeezed orange juice have considerably more vitamin C than juices made from concentrates. Citrus fruits, kiwis, strawberries, black currants, red, yellow, and green peppers, watercress, and freshly chopped parsley are very good sources of vitamin C. Green vegetables (savoy cabbage, curly kale, Brussels sprouts, broccoli, and watercress), red cabbage, and tomatoes are other good sources. Vitamin C is not stable when heated, so these vegetables are best eaten raw or after only light cooking. Vitamin C deficiency is quite common in elderly people eating calorie-rich, micronutrient-poor foods, and inadequate vitamin C consumption may be more common in the general population than is currently thought. Nosebleeds, bruising, frequent infections, slow healing of wounds, and poor gum health are indicators of vitamin C deficiency. Daily intake for adults should be 60 milligrams.

FOOD	SERVING SIZE	VITAMIN C (MG)
Kiwi	1 medium (3 ounces)	49
Red bell pepper	$1/_2$ medium (3 ounces)	140
Broccoli	3 ounces	47
Orange	1 medium (5 ounces)	75
Strawberries	3 ounces	58

FOODS RICH in minerals

The major minerals we need to consume on a daily basis are calcium, phosphorus, magnesium, potassium, sodium, and chloride. Sulphur is often mentioned as an essential mineral, but our needs are met by consumption of foods containing the sulphur amino acids methionine and cysteine; these are found in many protein foods from both animal and vegetable sources.

CALCIUM AND PHOSPHORUS are essential for healthy bones and teeth. Calcium is also involved in many cellular functions and helps to regulate blood pressure. Fish, particularly sardines and canned salmon, when the bones are eaten, are rich sources of calcium and phosphorus; cheese is another good source. Milk, yogurt, tofu, and tahini (sesame seed paste, used to make hummus) are good sources. Various seeds, nuts, fruits, vegetables, and pulses all contribute calcium to the overall daily intake.

Phosphorus is found in many of the same foods as calcium, so it is fairly easy to get a balanced intake of both. Phosphorus is involved in so many cellular functions that it is not conceivable to live without it. But this applies to every living thing, so phosphorus can be considered a ubiquitous mineral. Daily intake of calcium for adults should be 1000 milligrams; 1300 milligrams after the age of fifty.

FOOD	SERVING SIZE	CALCIUM (MG)
Canned sardines, with bones	2 ounces	249
Broccoli	3.5 ounces	40
Milk	1 cup (8 ounces)	285
Okra, boiled	3 ounces	84
Parmesan cheese	0.5 ounces	170

MAGNESIUM is essential for healthy nerves and muscles, and for strong bones. It is also necessary for a variety of cellular functions. Symptoms of magnesium deficiency include cramps and irregular heartbeat. Seeds, nuts, whole grains, pulses, vegetables, shellfish, and dried fruits are rich sources. Every natural food contains some magnesium. Daily intake of magnesium should be 270 milligrams for women, 300 milligrams for men.

FOOD	SERVING SIZE	MAGNESIUM (MG)
Pumpkin seeds	1 tablespoon (½ ounce)	75
Unsweetened cocoa powder	1 tablespoon	30
Crab	3 ounces	50
Quinoa	3.5 ounces	210
Red kidney beans	3 ounces	38

POTASSIUM is crucial for establishing equilibrium with sodium to regulate fluid balance. This is central to the function of every cell. Most foods contain some potassium, but eating plenty of potassium-rich foods—such as fresh and dried fruits, avocados, and nuts—helps counter the adverse effects of eating too much salt (sodium chloride). This can help lower blood pressure. Daily intake of potassium for adults should be 3500 milligrams.

CHLORIDE AND SODIUM, which everybody knows as salt, are important minerals, but most foods contain more than adequate amounts. As a general rule, adding extra salt to meals can put you at risk of high blood pressure.

Salt deficiency is generally unlikely. But in a very hot environment salt may be depleted through sweat. A potentially dangerous condition of low blood sodium levels called hyponatremia can occur, particularly if an individual drinks excessive amounts of water and sweats profusely. Night leg cramps may be a symptom of inadequate salt intake, but if you regularly suffer from leg cramps (unrelated to heavy sweating or hot weather), you should visit your doctor to exclude anything requiring treatment.

FOOD SOURCES OF TRACE ELEMENTS

With the exception of iron, trace element deficiencies are considered fairly rare. However, there may be an almost imperceptible difference between consuming just enough of a particular trace element to avoid symptoms of deficiency and having an increased likelihood of a disease because your daily intake is inadequate. Some research suggests levels of trace elements in food may be slowly declining because of intensive farming and the resulting depletion of soil sources. If this is true, it is hard to estimate at what point relative deficiencies of some trace elements may become a more important problem. This could be an argument for organic farming, but perhaps more importantly, it emphasizes the need for a varied diet of healthy foods so that a balanced intake of all vitamins and micronutrients is achieved.

IODINE Insufficient consumption is the classic example of trace element deficiency due to inadequate levels in the soil. It is still a problem in some parts of the world today. Iodine deficiency leads to insufficient thyroid hormone production, which results in mental retardation as well as various metabolic, developmental, and growth abnormalities. Farm animals reared on iodine-deficient soil may be prone to health problems, so salt licks are often provided.

Fish, shellfish, and seaweed are particularly rich sources; dairy foods, vegetables, and meat also contribute to our daily iodine intake. In most countries table salt includes added iodine (iodized salt). Sea salt often contains some iodine but in far smaller quantities. The advice to cut down on salt consumption may be increasing the risk of iodine deficiency in people who have relied on iodized salt for their iodine intake. Daily intake of iodine should be 110 micrograms for women, 130 micrograms for men.

IRON is an essential part of hemoglobin, the red pigment in blood that allows it to carry oxygen around the body. Anemia is the most common medical diagnosis of iron deficiency. Weakness, paleness, tiredness, and breathlessness are common symptoms of anemia.

Red meat, game, and liver are the best sources of iron. Clams are also a good source. The iron from animal sources is more readily absorbed by the body than the iron from vegetable sources such as pulses, sesame seeds, pumpkin seeds, flaxseeds, green leafy vegetables, and whole grains, including quinoa. Vitamin C helps iron absorption, so meals that combine dietary sources of iron with a source of vitamin C (such as fruits or bell peppers) will ensure best uptake. Polyphenols are reported to interfere with iron absorption, but I think it is unlikely that this interaction is sufficient to cause deficiencies in people consuming a healthy diet. Daily intake of iron should be 14.8 milligrams for women, 8.7 milligrams for men.

FOOD	SERVING SIZE	IRON (MG)
Lamb's liver, seared	3.5 ounces	10
Clams	2 ounces	16
Lentils, boiled	3.5 ounces	3.5
Spinach	3 ounces	2.4
Whole-wheat bread	2 slices (2.5 ounces)	2

SELENIUM is a good example of the fine balance that exists between getting just enough of a nutrient to avoid deficiency but not getting enough to protect against an increased risk of illness. Several studies have shown that low intakes of selenium increase the risk of cancer and heart disease. In countries where selenium levels in the soil were low there would be a likelihood of deficiency, but now that our food comes from a variety of countries, this

FOOD	SERVING SIZE	SELENIUM (MCG)
Brazil nuts	2 (⅛ ounce)	87
Sardines, canned in oil	3.5 ounces	50
Mussels	flesh only (2 ounces)	37
Whole-wheat pasta	5 ounces	23
Chicken breast, broiled	5 ounces	30

is less likely. Brazil nuts are the richest natural source of selenium—one or two Brazil nuts a day will meet all selenium requirements. Onions and garlic can be a good source because these vegetables are able to concentrate selenium from the soil. The more seafood, whole-grain foods, and vegetables you eat the less likely you are to be troubled by inadequate selenium consumption. Daily intake of selenium should be 60 micrograms for women, 75 micrograms for men.

ZINC plays an important role in many enzyme reactions and helps wounds to heal. Deficiency can lead to poor immune function and increased risk of infections. Zinc is abundant in liver and shellfish, particularly oysters. Nuts, seeds, pulses, and whole-grain, meat, poultry, and dairy foods are also good sources of zinc. Daily intake of zinc should be 7 milligrams for women, 9.5 milligrams for men.

FOOD	SERVING SIZE	ZINC (MG)
Oyster, raw	1 (flesh only), ⅛ ounce	5
Calves' liver	3 ounces	11
Pumpkin seeds	1 tablespoon (½ ounce)	1.1
Whole-wheat bread	2 slices (2.5 ounces)	1.3
Cheddar cheese	1 ounce	1.3

CHROMIUM deficiency has been linked to diabetes and heart disease, but its full physiological role has yet to be discovered. The ideal daily amount is also uncertain. Studies of chromium supplements in individuals with a mixed diet often show little benefit, so low chromium may be a marker of poor diet, rather than a major cause of these health problems. There is also concern over toxicity from excess chromium intake in supplement takers. Eggs, liver, meat, cheese, and vegetables are good sources of chromium.

COPPER is involved in many cellular functions, often acting in concert with iron and zinc. Because iron metabolism requires some copper, the cause of anemia sometimes can be traced to a deficiency in copper. However, it is a relatively common element and inadequate copper consumption is rare.

FLUORIDE, MANGANESE, AND MOLYBDENUM are other essential trace elements. These are fairly common elements, so with a varied diet we don't need to make a special effort to consume them. The importance of other trace elements such as boron and silicon is still uncertain, but a healthy mixed diet is likely to provide adequate intake for them, too.

encouraging good bacteria

Normal healthy intestines are full of bacteria, which are known as the gut flora; this develops from birth. Typically there are more than two pounds of live bacteria in the intestines at any one time. More than 100 different types of bacteria have been identified, although there may be as many as 400. The normal gut flora help prevent the growth of harmful bacteria and other microorganisms such as yeast. Normal gut bacteria are also involved in digestion and metabolism. Interactions between gut bacteria and their human hosts are not fully understood, but they are thought to reduce the risk of colon cancer by metabolizing or inactivating carcinogens. They may also influence the whole intestinal environment to reduce inflammation and decrease episodes of inflammatory bowel disease.

A number of factors affect gut flora: poor diet, antibiotics, food poisoning, and old age have all been linked with reduced levels of beneficial bacteria. Probiotics are living microorganisms that in sufficient quantities can provide nourishment for healthy symbiotic bacteria. Studies have shown that probiotics can help restore normal intestinal function after diarrhea. They may also reduce constipation in individuals who are prone to this problem. Whether probiotics are of any value to healthy individuals is still an open question.

Probiotics are most commonly found in yogurt and probiotic drinks. Yogurt is fermented milk made with lactic acid–producing bacteria. Traditionally *Lactobacillus acidophilus* and *Streptococcus thermophilus* are used, but much emphasis in recent years has been placed on using *Bifidus* species. The ability of these bacteria to tolerate stomach acid is important if living bacteria are to reach the intestines. *Bifidobacterium longum* tolerates gastric acid better than some other *Bifidus* strains. Some of the commercially available probiotic drinks are based on strains of *Lactobacillus casei*, which also tolerates stomach acidity. These bacteria bind to the walls of the small and large intestines and prevent harmful bacteria from binding. *Lactobacilli* also stimulate secretion of protective antibodies, called immunoglobulin A, in the small intestine. This is a key defense mechanism to prevent infection by harmful bacteria.

My view is that natural yogurt is a healthy eating option, and if it has a probiotic effect, then that is simply a bonus. The best yogurts have nothing added except cultures of bacteria to start the fermentation. Natural yogurt with no added sugar contains around 5 grams of sugar per 100 grams. Look at the nutrition information on the label to check that it has not been sweetened with added sugar. I consider the fat content of yogurt irrelevant; a serving (3½ ounces) of whole milk yogurt contains around 3 grams of fat. As part of a healthy diet, with limited meat consumption, this is an insignificant amount of fat.

Some probiotic drinks are marketed with the promise that they will make you feel good. The ones I have seen contain a lot of sugar, so any pick-you-up effect is likely to be the result of a sugar rush. Capsules containing specific bacteria can also have a probiotic effect, but the quality of products is inconsistent.

Prebiotics are indigestible carbohydrates, particularly fructo- and galacto-oligosaccharides, which pass through to the large intestine where the gut flora can digest them by fermentation. Prebiotics are a source of nutrients for healthy bacteria and may be just as important as probiotics for promoting their growth and encouraging their protective effects. Jerusalem artichokes, asparagus, leeks, and onions are good sources of prebiotics.

THE PROMISE OF DIETARY PHYTOESTROGENS

Much has been written on the benefits of increased soy consumption. The principal argument for soy comes from studies in Asia that have shown lower heart disease and fewer cancers of the breast, endometrium, and prostate in people who eat soy-based foods as a key component of their diet. Diets rich in soy products may also help reduce osteoporosis. Although there is extensive evidence to support these beneficial effects, patient and volunteer studies have often failed to reveal the same benefits.

An explanation for these disappointing outcomes has come from studies of the metabolism of isoflavones (isoflavones are the active phytoestrogens in soybeans). Equol seems to be the molecule responsible for many of the beneficial effects of soy phytoestrogens, but only 20 to 35 percent of people are able to metabolize the abundant soy isoflavone daidzein into equol. The reason equol is produced only in some people is a bit of mystery, but it appears to depend on their intestinal flora. It is not yet known which bacteria are responsible, so there is not yet a probiotic product that can convert nonproducers into producers. Dietary prebiotics (fructo-oligosaccharides) may also be important if the equol-synthesizing bacteria are to thrive in the intestines. This lack of "equolity" explains why some individuals will gain more from soy products than others. Nevertheless, eating soy is an important way of boost vegetable protein intake, and greater consumption of vegetable protein is in itself linked to better health.

COMPLETE NUTRITION—THE REAL POLYMEAL

While I was working on this book a tongue-in-cheek article was published in the Christmas 2004 issue of the *British Medical Journal* in response to a previous article that suggested the development of a medicine called the Polypill. (The Polypill is a concept of combining different medications into a single pill, which could in theory be administered to everyone over fifty-five to cut heart disease and stroke by 80 to 90 percent.) The authors of the 2004 article, having examined the evidence for the protective effects from regular consumption of various foods and drinks, proposed the Polymeal as a nutritious alternative to medical therapies for reducing heart disease and increasing life expectancy. Here's what was on the menu:

- Wine, 5 ounces a day
- Fish, 4 ounces four times a week

- Fruits and vegetables, 14 ounces a day
- Garlic, 1 clove a day
- Dark chocolate, 3.5 ounces a day
- Almonds, 2.5 ounces a day

From their analysis of published research the authors concluded that a lifestyle including these foods and drinks could reduce heart disease by 76 percent and extend life expectancy by 6.6 years for men and 4.8 years for women. These recommendations are a logical progression from diet research, and I was surprised at the subsequent dismissive and humorless correspondence published by the *British Medical Journal* on this article.

In many respects my approach is similar: I have drawn conclusions from diet research and in this book I have looked at the ideal combination of nutrients, with an emphasis on the best choices. Wine, fish, fruit, vegetables, and garlic are already part of a healthy Mediterranean diet. To maximize the benefits, I recommend a careful choice of wine (see Chapter 7). Eating a variety of fruits and vegetables throughout the week is important so that all vitamins and minerals are covered. At least one portion of polyphenol-rich fruits (such as apples, cranberries, pomegranates, or raspberries) every day is likely to be beneficial (see Chapter 4). The amount of chocolate recommended in the Polymeal is too much from a calorie point of view (approximately 500 to 600 calories). Procyanidin-rich dark chocolate would be best,

---

WHERE TO CUT CALORIES

If you keep to simple goals, weight loss will happen gradually and naturally. Cutting out 200 calories a day eventually will make a difference.

· *pint of beer*	*190 calories*
· *bagel, croissant, or scone*	*200 to 300 calories*
· *popcorn (3.5 ounces)*	*400 calories*
· *small bag (1.5 ounces) of potato chips*	*190 calories*
· *medium to large potato*	*250 calories*
· *small portion of French fries*	*300 calories*

---

as only about 1 ounce is needed to gain the benefit. Walnuts—which contain both protective polyphenols and a high proportion of omega-3 fats—are probably a better choice than almonds, but variety is a good idea. My food and drink recommendations in this chapter and in the sample weekly menus and recipes that follow are the real Polymeal.

GETTING DOWN TO DIETING

You probably know if you are overweight: the Body Mass Index charts at the end of this book will give you a clearer idea of a healthy weight for your height. To lose weight, the number of calories you eat needs to be less than the amount your body uses in your daily routine. Many people follow a weight loss diet until they reach their target weight, and then put the weight back on. Unless you change the way you eat and start to exercise, you are not going to see a permanent loss of body fat nor will you make a long-term improvement in health.

My two-week sample meal plan (see pages 217 to 221) is designed to get you into the habit of eating healthier food. If you want to lose weight, meals have to be satisfying so that you do not resort to too many between-meal snacks. Cutting out refined starchy foods and sugary foods and drinks will actually help curb cravings. Getting regular exercise and eating at the times of day that suit you best will benefit your overall health and well-being. You might find that these changes in diet and lifestyle also result in gradual weight loss over the course of a few months. If not, then controlling portion size is the next step rather than giving up particular foods.

If you don't cook, learn how to prepare simple and nutritious meals (see the recipe section and menu plan for some ideas to start with). This is the best way to avoid the excess sugar, salt, and refined and overprocessed starches and fats found in ready-made foods. You may be surprised to find that after cooking a meal your appetite is reduced; this can help you lose weight. And most important, make a meal of it; food should not be stuffed in at a hasty pit stop but enjoyed slowly to avoid taking in excess calories.

The keys to weight loss are the same as those for improving health and quality of life:

- Eat a variety of fruits and vegetables.
- Reduce meat consumption, replacing it with vegetable protein sources, particularly beans and pulses and more fish.
- Increase consumption of whole-grain foods.
- Cut out refined starchy products.
- Cut out foods and drinks with added sugar.
- Reduce saturated fat intake and replace with foods rich in monounsaturated fats and polyunsaturated fats (particularly omega-3 fats).
- Never eat foods containing hydrogenated fats (trans fats).
- Reduce salt intake.
- Drink wine mainly with meals, and refrain from excessive consumption.

a two-week sample menu plan

Each day's meals provide between 1400 and 2000 calories. An apple a day adds about 70 calories. A 4-ounce glass of red wine, a 1-ounce piece of dark chocolate, or a piece of the Cranberry and Walnut Bars (page 229) or Fruity Oat Bars (page 230) will add 150 to 200 calories. Apart from fruits—or vegetables such as cherry tomatoes, carrots, celery or peppers—I do not recommend snacking between meals, especially if you are trying to lose weight; a break between meals allows your body to enter fat-burning mode. However, if you skip breakfast, have a midmorning snack of a no-added-sugar bar (pages 229 to 230), or fruits or vegetables, plus some plain yogurt or cottage cheese; flavor with cinnamon or herbs if you like.

This menu plan is low in saturated fat; the emphasis is on monounsaturated fats, like the original healthy Mediterranean diet. To ensure a good intake of omega-3 polyunsaturated fat; keep a bottle of flaxseed oil in the fridge and sprinkle 1 teaspoon over salads and vegetables; eat oily fish two or three times a week; choose grass-fed beef and lamb and free-range poultry; and eat plenty of green vegetables.

Monday

BREAKFAST

Slice of Four-seed Bread
(page 227), toasted,
with Cranberry
and Orange Compote
(page 225)

LUNCH

Avocado, tuna, and white
beans with salad greens
and vinaigrette
Kiwi and raspberries

DINNER

Shrimp and Peanut
Stir-fry (page 261)
Brown rice
Steamed bok choy
or broccoli

Tuesday

BREAKFAST

Muesli (page 224)
with milk, grated
apple, and dried
cranberries

LUNCH

Lentil, Spinach, and
Feta Cheese Salad
(page 244)
6 ounces plain yogurt
Peach or nectarine

DINNER

Salmon with Watercress-
Tofu Sauce (page 257)
Baked tomatoes
New potatoes boiled in
their skins, green beans

Wednesday

BREAKFAST

Fruity Oat Bar (page 230)
6 ounces plain yogurt with
1 tablespoon sunflower
seeds
Cranberry juice

LUNCH

Smoked Fish and
Tofu Pâté (page 235)
Slice of whole-wheat bread
Carrot and Parsley Salad
with Pomegranate
Vinaigrette (page 241)
Watercress salad

DINNER

Stir-fried Liver
(page 273)
Brown rice
Steamed kale
or broccoli, sprinkled
with 1 teaspoon
sesame oil

Thursday

BREAKFAST

Poached egg
Slice of Four-Seed Bread
(page 227)
Pomegranate juice

LUNCH

Chicken, Orange, and
Fennel Salad (page 246)
Raspberries, blueberries,
strawberries

DINNER

Spaghetti with Walnut
and Eggplant Sauce
(page 255)
Arugula, watercress, and
spinach salad

Friday

BREAKFAST
Pomegranate, pear, and kiwi salad
6 ounces plain yogurt with 1 tablespoon mixed seeds

LUNCH
Broiled sardines (canned or fresh)
Tomato salad with basil and vinaigrette
Slice of whole-wheat bread

DINNER
Collard Green Loaf with Spicy Tomato Sauce (page 253)
Carrots, potatoes
Chocolate Truffle "Ice Cream" (page 274) with raspberries

Saturday

BREAKFAST
Muesli (page 224) with milk, grated pear, and cinnamon

LUNCH
Greek Salad
6 ounces plain yogurt with fresh figs or passion fruit

DINNER
Monkfish Kebabs with Pomegranate Salsa (page 259)
Tabbouleh (page 252)
Lima bean purée

Sunday

BREAKFAST
½ grapefruit
Sliced tomato and lean bacon
Slice of Walnut Bread (page 226)

LUNCH
Spaghetti with Tomato and Anchovy Sauce (page 256)
Grapes

DINNER
Leeks with Cranberry Vinaigrette (page 240)
Spicy Chicken Mole (page 265)
Quinoa, mixed salad

Monday

BREAKFAST
Muesli (page 224) with milk and yogurt
Raspberries, blueberries, strawberries

LUNCH
Broiled sardines (canned or fresh)
Fava bean and Pea Purée (page 250)
Arugula and romaine lettuce salad

DINNER
Lentil, Bacon, and Cabbage Soup (page 231)
Slice of Walnut Bread (page 226)
Cottage cheese

Tuesday

BREAKFAST
Fruity Oat Bar
 (page 230)
6 ounces plain yogurt
Cranberry juice

LUNCH
Tomato salad
Spicy Chickpea and
 Apricot Pâté (page 237)
Pita bread
Grated carrot, chopped
 red pepper, ½ head
 romaine lettuce

DINNER
Faisanjin (Chicken with
 Pomegranates and
 Walnuts) (page 267)
Middle Eastern–style
 Vegetables (page 268)
Brown rice

Wednesday

BREAKFAST
Muesli (page 224) with
 milk, dried fruit, and
 grated apple

LUNCH
Avocado, tomato, and
 mozzarella salad
Slice of Soya and
 Flaxseed Bread
 (page 227)

DINNER
Salmon with Rye and
 Kidney Beans
 (page 258)
Italian-style Mixed
 Greens (page 248)

Thursday

BREAKFAST
Peach or nectarine
Slice of Walnut Bread
 (page 226) with
 1 tablespoon
 unsweetened peanut
 butter

LUNCH
Salade Niçoise
 (page 247)
6 ounces plain yogurt
 with raspberries
1 tablespoon
 sunflower seeds

DINNER
Bean and Tomato
 Casserole (page 249)
Green beans, asparagus
Chocolate Truffle
 "Ice Cream"
 (page 274)

Friday

BREAKFAST
Cranberry and
 Walnut Bar (page 229)
Fresh fruit juice

LUNCH
Mushroom and Lentil
 Pâté (page 236) with
 raw vegetables
Slice of whole-wheat toast
6 ounces plain yogurt
1 kiwi

DINNER
Fava Bean Soup with
 Scallions and Mint
 (page 234)
Broiled Mackerel with
 Beet and Cranberry
 Salad (page 262)
Bulgur wheat
Watercress salad

Saturday

BREAKFAST	LUNCH	DINNER
½ grapefruit	Grilled chicken	Nut Roast (page 254)
1 poached egg	Roasted Bell Peppers	with Spicy Tomato
Sautéed mushrooms	with Anchovies	Sauce (page 253)
and tomato	(page 238)	Italian-style Mixed
Slice of whole-	Arugula and	Greens (page 248)
wheat toast	avocado salad	Baked apple with
		dried fruit, cinnamon,
		and yogurt

Sunday

BREAKFAST	LUNCH	DINNER
Slice of melon	Bean Soup with	Beef Stew with
Rye and Cranberry Bread	Olives (page 233)	Cranberries (page 271)
(page 228) with	served with pesto	Broccoli, new potatoes
cottage cheese		6 ounces plain yogurt
Fresh fruit juice		with mixed berries

recipes

Everyday Muesli

I make a batch of the basic mix every week. It's easy to dip into and there are any number of variations (see below).

SERVES 10

1 cup oat flakes or rolled oats	*5 tablespoons sunflower seeds*
1 cup barley flakes or rolled barley	*7 tablespoons chopped Brazil nuts*
1 cup rye flakes or rolled rye	*10 dried figs, chopped*
5 tablespoons pumpkin seeds	*20 prunes, chopped*

MIX all the ingredients together and store in a sealed container in a cool place.

To serve, spoon 4 tablespoons of muesli into a bowl. Add 1 tablespoon freshly ground flaxseed. Add ⅔ cup milk, soy milk, or unsweetened apple juice and mix well. Top with 1 tablespoon yogurt.

VARIATIONS

Oats are the basis for muesli, but I usually include one or two other grains from my local health food store. Instead of barley or rye, you could try millet or quinoa.

- Add dried fruits: chopped dried apricots, dates, apples, pears
- Add fresh fruits: grated apple or pear, halved grapes, banana, strawberries, raspberries, blackberries, blueberries
- Add nuts: chopped walnuts, flaked almonds, hazelnuts, pecans
- Add spice: ground cinnamon or freshly grated nutmeg

NUTRITIONAL BENEFITS

With no added sugar and plenty of fiber, this muesli is also a good source of B vitamins and minerals, such as zinc and iron. One serving provides your body with half its daily magnesium and nearly a third of its daily calcium requirements. One or two Brazil nuts a day contain all the selenium you need.

Per serving (with skim milk and yogurt): 18g protein, 60g carbohydrate, 15g fat, 11g fiber, 422 calories/1776 kJ

One or two servings of fresh fruit, particularly berries and citrus fruits, is always a good start to the day. The following choices weigh approximately 3 ounces, which constitutes one of the recommended daily five to nine servings:

1 apple, pear, orange, nectarine, or peach

2 or 3 fresh apricots or plums

1 small to medium banana

berries: weigh them to get 3-ounce servings

20 cherries or grapes

2 clementines or tangerines

1 or 2 fresh figs or kiwis

half a grapefruit, mango, or small papaya

small slice of canteloupe or watermelon

If you have a juicer, make some fruit or vegetable juice using fresh or frozen fruit. It won't have the fiber content of the fresh fruit, but you'll get a good helping of vitamins and minerals. Try apple, carrot, and ginger; cranberry, strawberry, and blueberry; or orange, strawberry, and peach.

Cranberry and Orange Compote

This compote is delicious stirred into yogurt for breakfast, and is equally good on toast or as a sauce to accompany roast turkey, pork, or game.

SERVES 3

1 cup fresh or frozen cranberries

1 tablespoons fresh orange juice, or more if needed

2 teaspoons honey, or to taste

COOK the cranberries in the orange juice, in a medium saucepan over low heat for 6 to 7 minutes, until soft, adding more orange juice if needed to keep the cranberries moist. Add honey to taste. Serve with plain yogurt.

NUTRITIONAL BENEFITS

A serving of this compote with ½ cup plain yogurt provides a good balance of carbs, fats, and protein; it also makes a useful contribution to your daily vitamin C and calcium requirements. Lightly cooked cranberries are a good source of procyanidins—a serving of this compote gives you just slightly fewer procyanidins than a 4-ounce glass of procyanidin-rich red wine.

Per serving (with yogurt): 4g protein, 13g carbohydrate, 3g fat, 2g fiber, 91 calories/380 kJ

WALNUT BREAD

Modern breadmaking machines make it really easy to wake up to freshly baked bread. I've developed some healthy variations on the all-in-one method.

MAKES 1 LOAF (16 SLICES)

1⅓ cups white bread flour

1⅔ cups whole-wheat flour

1¼ cup soy flour

1¾ teaspoons instant yeast for breadmaking machines

1 teaspoon dark brown sugar

½ teaspoon salt

¼ teaspoon vitamin C (ascorbic acid) powder

1 tablespoon walnut oil

⅔ cup soy milk

1¼ cups warm water

1¼ cups chopped walnuts

MIX all the flours together in a large bowl, then place all the ingredients in the breadmaking machine and follow the manufacturer's instructions.

ALTERNATIVELY, to make the bread by hand, use 1 package active dry yeast, omit the vitamin C powder, and reduce the water to ⅔ cup. Stir the flours, yeast, sugar, and salt together in a large bowl. Add the walnut oil, soy milk, and warm water, mix well, then knead for about 15 minutes, until the dough is springy; work in a little more flour if the dough sticks to your fingers. Cover and leave in a warm place to double in size (about 1 hour).

KNEAD the dough again; add the walnuts and work them into the dough. Put the dough into a large loaf pan, cover with lightly oiled plastic wrap, and leave to rise again (30 to 45 minutes).

PREHEAT the oven to 425°F. When the dough has risen to almost fill the pan, remove the plastic wrap, place in the oven, and bake for about 30 minutes. Test by turning out the bread and knocking on the base with your knuckles. If the bread is done it will sound hollow; if not, return it to the oven for 5 or 10 minutes.

VARIATIONS

⊛ Four-Seed Bread: Replace the walnuts with 5 tablespoons flaxseeds and 1 tablespoon each of sunflower seeds, pumpkin seeds, and sesame seeds.

⊛ Soy and Flaxseed Bread: Replace the walnuts with ⅔ cup flaxseeds. This variation has an ideal 1 to 1 ratio of omega-3 to omega-6 fats.

⊛ Flaxseed and Hemp Bread: Replace the walnuts with 5 tablespoons flaxseeds and 5 tablespoons hemp seeds, ground together in a coffee grinder.

NUTRITIONAL BENEFITS

Adding soy flour, nuts, and seeds makes any bread nutritionally more complete, and it reduces the glycemic load of a slice of bread.

Per slice: 7g protein, 22g carbohydrate, 7g fat, 3g fiber, 168 calories/706 kJ

Rye and Cranberry Bread

Most of the cranberries in this loaf will remain whole and burst juicily in your mouth when you bite into them. It's lovely while still warm from the oven, or toasted, with butter, honey, or cheese.

MAKES 1 SMALL LOAF (12 SLICES)

1 tablespoon active dry yeast

1 teaspoon dark brown sugar

about ⅔ cup warm water

3 tablespoons extra-virgin olive oil

½ teaspoon salt

1⅔ cups whole-wheat bread flour

1 cup rye flour

⅔ cup rye flakes or rolled rye

1¼ cups fresh cranberries

5 tablespoons sunflower seeds

PUT the yeast, sugar, and warm water in a large bowl. Stir to mix and leave in a warm place for about 10 minutes, until frothy.

ADD the oil, salt, flours, and flakes. Mix well and then knead for about 15 minutes. The dough should be springy and not sticky; work in a little more flour if it sticks to your fingers or the bowl. Cover the bowl with plastic wrap and leave in a warm place until it has doubled in size (about 2 hours).

KNEAD the dough again; add the cranberries and sunflower seeds and work them into the dough. Put the dough into a small loaf pan, cover with lightly oiled plastic wrap, and leave to rise again (about 45 minutes).

PREHEAT the oven to 425°F. When the dough has risen to almost fill the pan, remove the plastic wrap, place in the oven, and bake for about 30 minutes. Test by turning out the bread and knocking on the base with your knuckles: if the bread is done it will sound hollow; if not, return it to the oven for 5 or 10 minutes.

NUTRITIONAL BENEFITS

As the cranberries remain whole in this loaf, they retain most of their procyanidins, even though they are cooked for 30 minutes. Like most whole-grain breads, this is a good source of fiber.

Per slice: 5g protein, 26g carbohydrate, 6g fat, 5g fiber, 170 calories/712 kJ

Cranberry and Walnut Bars

━━━

This recipe and the next make great breakfasts or snacks.

MAKES 16 BARS

1 cup soy flour

⅔ cup whole-wheat self-rising flour

2 teaspoons ground cinnamon

Grated zest and juice of 2 large oranges

2 large eggs (preferably omega-3 rich)

1 tablespoon walnut oil

1¾ cups roughly chopped walnuts

½ cup chopped almonds

⅔ cup chopped dried figs

⅔ cup chopped dried dates

1½ cups fresh or frozen cranberries, or scant 1 cup dried cranberries

PREHEAT the oven to 350°F. Line an 8-inch square baking pan with parchment paper.

MIX the flours and cinnamon together in a large bowl. Add the orange zest. Gently whisk the eggs with the oil, add the orange juice, then stir into the flour and mix well. Add the nuts and fruits. Spoon the mixture into the pan and bake for 45 minutes.

WHILE still hot, cut into 16 portions. Allow to cool completely before removing from the baking pan. Store in a sealed container in the refrigerator.

NUTRITIONAL BENEFITS

With no added sugar, and a low glycemic load, these bars are far better for you than most of those you can buy. Cinnamon and cranberries are good sources of procyanidins and walnuts contain other beneficial polyphenols.

Per bar: 6g protein, 17g carbohydrate, 12g fat, 4g fiber, 190 calories/800 kJ

Fruity Oat Bars

Cold-pressed canola oil is available from health food stores; buy small bottles so you can keep it in the refrigerator.

makes 16 bars

*1 pound apples (weight after
    peeling and coring), grated*
Juice of 1 lemon or 2 limes
2 tablespoons water
⅔ cup rolled oats
*⅔ cup whole-wheat self-
    rising flour*

1 tablespoon canola oil
2 teaspoons vanilla extract (optional)
¾ cup chopped Brazil nuts
¾ cup chopped hazelnuts
¾ cup chopped dried apricots
1¼ cups dried cranberries
5 tablespoons pumpkin seeds

PREHEAT the oven to 350°F. Line an 8-inch square baking pan with parchment paper.

PUT the grated apple, lemon juice, and water in a nonstick saucepan, cover, and cook gently for a few minutes, until soft. Remove from the heat and stir in the oats, flour, oil, and vanilla, and leave to stand for 10 minutes so that the oats absorb the liquid.

ADD the nuts, fruits, and seeds, and stir well. Spoon the mixture into the pan and bake for 55 to 60 minutes.

WHILE still hot, cut into 16 portions. Allow to cool completely before removing from the baking pan. Store in a sealed container in the refrigerator.

NUTRITIONAL BENEFITS

Apples and cranberries are good sources of procyanidins to boost your daily intake. The fruits provide both sweetness (no added sugar) and fiber, and the nuts and seeds contribute vitamin E and minerals—selenium in particular, but also magnesium and a small amount of iron.

Per bar: 5g protein, 26g carbohydrate, 11g fat, 4g fiber, 205 calories/860 kJ

Lentil, Bacon, and Cabbage Soup

This chunky soup is a meal in itself—with a glass of red wine, of course.

serves 4

1 tablespoon extra-virgin olive oil

2 ounces sliced bacon, rind
   removed, chopped

2 onions, finely chopped

2 carrots, finely chopped

4 cloves garlic, crushed

¾ cup green lentils,
   thoroughly washed

One 14-ounce can chopped tomatoes

4 cups fresh stock or water

Salt and freshly ground black pepper

3 cups shredded savoy cabbage

HEAT the oil in a large saucepan over low heat. Add the bacon, onions, carrots, and garlic, and cook for 5 minutes, or until the vegetables soften. Add the lentils, tomatoes, and stock; bring to a boil, then reduce the heat and simmer for 40 minutes, or until the lentils have softened.

TASTE and season with salt and pepper, then add the cabbage and simmer for an additional 5 to 10 minutes, until the cabbage is just tender. Serve at once.

THE lentil soup can be made a day ahead, covered, and refrigerated—but do not add the seasoning or cabbage until the soup is reheated.

NUTRITIONAL BENEFITS

A bowl of this soup provides a generous two servings of vegetables toward the recommended five to nine a day. It's packed with healthy carotenoids (including lutein and zeaxanthin), vitamin C, and folate, along with other B vitamins and minerals and plenty of fiber.

Per serving: 13g protein, 38g carbohydrate, 10g fat, 15g fiber, 281 calories/1180 kJ

Winter Vegetable Soup

*For a quick and easy vegetable stock I use vegetable bouillon powder.
A teaspoon of flaxseed oil swirled into the soup adds valuable omega-3 fats
and a nutty flavor. The soup can be made a day ahead—add the parsley and
flaxseed oil just before serving.*

SERVES 4

1 tablespoon extra-virgin olive oil	*Salt and freshly ground*
1 onion, chopped	*black pepper*
1½ cups chopped carrots	*4 cups vegetable stock or water*
1 garlic clove, chopped	*2 tablespoons chopped*
3 cups chopped savoy cabbage	*fresh parsley*
14 ounces Jerusalem artichokes	*4 teaspoons flaxseed oil*
(sunchokes), peeled and chopped	

HEAT the olive oil in a large saucepan over low heat. Add the onion and carrots and cook until they begin to soften, about 5 minutes. Add the garlic, cabbage, artichokes, and a pinch of salt, stir well, then cook for 10 minutes to release the juices.

ADD the stock, stir well, bring to a boil, then reduce the heat and simmer for about 20 minutes, or until the vegetables are tender. Transfer to a blender and purée. Return the soup to the pan, then season with salt and pepper to taste. Reheat gently and serve hot, with each bowl sprinkled with parsley and 1 teaspoon flaxseed oil.

NUTRITIONAL BENEFITS

Each bowl of soup provides a generous two servings of vegetables toward your daily five to nine recommended servings. There are plenty of carotenoids, vitamin C, and iron—and Jerusalem artichokes are a good source of prebiotics, which encourage healthy bacteria in the gut.

Per serving: 4g protein, 28g carbohydrate, 9g fat, 5g fiber, 197 calories/827 kJ

Bean Soup with Olives

This is a variation on the Provençal vegetable soup known as soupe au pistou; *you could do as they do in the south of France and swirl in a spoonful of pesto just before serving.*

serves 4

½ cup dried cannellini or
    kidney beans, soaked for at least
    6 hours or overnight (or two
    14-ounce cans, drained)
1 tablespoon extra-virgin olive oil
1 onion, diced
1 carrot, diced
2 celery stalks, chopped
2 cloves garlic, crushed
4 ounces green beans, cut into
    1-inch lengths

1 zucchini, sliced
1 tablespoon tomato purée
2 to 3 sprigs of basil, or 2 teaspoons
    dried mixed herbs (herbes
    de Provence)
Salt and freshly ground
    black pepper
3½ cups vegetable stock
7 ounces fresh spinach,
    shredded
¼ cup pitted olives, halved

DRAIN the soaked beans, place in a large saucepan, cover with cold water—do not add salt—and bring to a boil. Boil for 10 minutes, then drain and rinse under cold water. Return to the pan, cover with cold water, bring to a boil, then reduce the heat and simmer for about 50 minutes, or until tender but not mushy. Drain.

HEAT the oil in the saucepan over low heat. Add the onion, carrot, and celery, and cook until they begin to soften, about 5 minutes. Add the garlic, cooked or canned beans, green beans, zucchini, tomato purée, herbs, and salt and pepper to taste. Add the stock, bring to a boil, then reduce the heat and simmer for 20 to 30 minutes, or until the vegetables are tender.

TASTE and adjust the seasonings if necessary. Add the shredded spinach and bring back to a boil for 2 to 3 minutes, until the spinach is wilted. Stir in the olives and serve hot.

Fava Bean Soup with Scallions and Mint

This early-summer soup should be made with fresh young fava beans, before the skins get tough. If you are using older beans, increase the quantity and first cook them for 2 to 3 minutes in boiling water, then drain and run cold water over them to cool. Peel off the skins so you are left with bright green beans.

SERVES 4

1 tablespoon extra-virgin olive oil

6 scallions, chopped, plus extra to garnish

1 clove garlic, chopped

5 cups shelled fava beans (fresh or frozen)

4 cups vegetable or chicken stock

3 tablespoons chopped fresh parsley

3 tablespoons chopped fresh mint, plus extra to garnish

Salt and freshly ground black pepper

1 ounce Pecorino Romano cheese, cut into flakes, to garnish

HEAT the oil in a large saucepan over low heat. Add the scallions and garlic and cook for 5 minutes, until softened but not browned. Add the beans and stock, bring to a boil, then reduce the heat and simmer for 7 to 8 minutes, until the beans are tender.

ADD the parsley, mint, and salt and pepper to taste. Transfer to a blender and purée. Return the soup to the pot, taste, and adjust the seasoning. Reheat gently and serve hot, garnished with mint leaves, scallions, and flakes of Pecorino cheese.

Beans, scallions, and herbs combine to make a generous serving of vegetables that is rich in folate and a good source of other B vitamins, vitamins A and C, and iron.

Per serving: 15g protein, 29g carbohydrate, 7g fat, 1g fiber, 202 calories/ 848 kJ

Smoked Fish and Tofu Pâté

Use smoked mackerel, trout, or salmon for variety in this easy-to-make pâté. To serve as a first course, decorate with a sprig of dill or some thinly sliced scallions and serve with lemon wedges.

serves 4

7 ounces smoked fish fillets　　　　**Juice of ½ lemon**
4 ounces silken tofu　　　　**Freshly ground black pepper to taste**

Place all the ingredients in a food processor and blend until smooth. You shouldn't need to add salt because the fish will be salty enough.

Store, covered, in the refrigerator for up to 2 days. Serve with whole-wheat toast or raw vegetables such as carrots, celery, and red and yellow bell peppers.

NUTRITIONAL BENEFITS

This pâté is high in healthy omega-3 fatty acids and is a good source of protein and vitamin B$_{12}$. Whole-wheat toast and/or raw vegetables will make this a nutritionally complete lunchtime snack.

Per serving: 11g protein, 1g carbohydrate, 3g fat, 0g fiber, 76 calories/318 kJ

Mushroom and Lentil Pâté

▨▨▨▨▨▨▨▨▨▨▨▨▨▨▨▨▨▨▨▨▨▨▨▨▨▨▨▨▨▨▨▨▨▨▨▨

This vegetarian pâté has quite a meaty taste, which will be even more pronounced if you use shiitake or porcini mushrooms. You can garnish with sprigs of fresh parsley or cilantro and lemon wedges if you like.

SERVES 4

1 small onion, quartered

2 cloves garlic, crushed

1 tablespoon extra-virgin olive oil

7 ounces fresh mushrooms, cleaned

¾ cup cooked or canned lentils

1 tablespoon soy sauce
  (preferably tamari)

1 tablespoon tomato purée

Freshly ground black pepper

1 tablespoon chopped fresh
  tarragon

Squeeze of lemon juice
  (optional)

PUT the onion and garlic in a food processor and chop finely. Heat the oil in a large saucepan over low heat, add the onion mixture, and cook until softened, about 5 minutes. Meanwhile, chop the mushrooms in the food processor; add to the softened onion, increase the heat to medium, and cook the mushrooms for 2 to 3 minutes, or until softened.

ADD the lentils, soy sauce, tomato purée, pepper to taste, and tarragon and cook for 5 minutes, mashing the lentils with a wooden spoon. Taste and adjust the seasoning, adding a squeeze of lemon juice if you like.

STORE, covered, in the refrigerator for up to 3 days. Serve with whole-wheat toast or carrot and celery sticks.

NUTRITIONAL BENEFITS

This pâté counts as one serving of vegetables; it's also a good source of B vitamins, particularly riboflavin, niacin, and folate, and it contains some iron.

Per serving: 6g protein, 12g carbohydrate, 4g fat, 4g fiber, 100 calories/420 kJ

Spicy Chickpea and Apricot Pâté

To add contrasting color and texture to this pâté, instead of processing the apricots, stir them into the puréed chickpeas.

serves 6

One 14-ounce can organic
   chickpeas, drained
⅓ cup dried apricots,
   roughly chopped
2 tablespoons tomato purée
1½ tablespoons extra-virgin
   olive oil
7 ounces silken tofu
Juice of ½ lemon

1 clove garlic, crushed
1 onion, chopped
½ teaspoon ground coriander
½ teaspoon ground cumin
½ teaspoon crushed dried
   chiles or cayenne pepper
½ teaspoon paprika
Salt (optional)

Place all the ingredients in a food processor and blend to a coarse purée. Taste and add more lemon juice, spices, or a little salt if you like.

Store, covered, in the refrigerator for up to 2 days. Serve with whole-wheat toast or stuff into whole-wheat pita bread with salad greens.

NUTRITIONAL BENEFITS
This vegetarian pâté contributes small amounts of a wide range of vitamins and minerals, particularly vitamin B_6. It also counts as a serving of vegetables.

Per serving: 5g protein, 20g carbohydrate, 5g fat, 3g fiber, 139 calories/584 kJ

Seville-style Chickpeas with Spinach

Almost all the tapas bars in Seville make some sort of variation on this theme. Saffron is expensive, but it will keep for several years in an airtight container.

2 tablespoons extra-virgin olive oil
4 cloves garlic, crushed
2 small dried chiles
1 teaspoon cumin seeds
Two 14-ounce cans chickpeas,
   drained

A good pinch of saffron, infused
   in a little boiling water
1 pound fresh spinach, washed
2 tablespoons good red wine
   or sherry vinegar
Salt and freshly ground black pepper

HEAT the oil in a large saucepan over low heat. Add the garlic, chiles, and cumin and cook for 5 minutes, or until the garlic is softened. Add the chickpeas and saffron. Remove the chiles after a minute or two. Add the spinach and the vinegar and cook 3 to 5 minutes, stirring occasionally, until the spinach is soft and most of the liquid has evaporated. Season with salt and pepper to taste and let stand for 30 minutes for the flavors to intensify. Serve at room temperature or cold.

NUTRITIONAL BENEFITS

The combination of chickpeas and spinach counts as two servings of vegetables. This dish is an excellent source of carotenoids, folate, and vitamins B_6 and K. It also provides more than half your daily vitamin C and a quarter of your iron and magnesium, along with other vitamins and minerals.

Per serving: 9g protein, 32g carbohydrate, 9g fat, 8g fiber, 234 calories/985 kJ

Roasted Bell Peppers with anchovies

Serve as an accompaniment to grilled fish, with brown rice or new potatoes. Alternatively, serve as part of a selection of tapas, or a first course or lunch, with a slice of Four-Seed Bread (see page 227) and green salad.

serves 4

2 large red bell peppers, cut in
   half lengthwise and seeded
20 cherry tomatoes, cut in half
2 cloves garlic, chopped

1 tablespoon extra-virgin olive oil
Freshly ground black pepper
One 2-ounce can anchovy
   fillets (8 fillets)

Preheat the oven to 350°F. Fill the halved bell peppers with the halved tomatoes. Sprinkle with the garlic, oil, and black pepper to taste. Snip 2 anchovy fillets over each half pepper. Place in a shallow roasting tray and bake near the top of the oven for about 1 hour, or until soft and slightly brown. Serve warm or cold.

NUTRITIONAL BENEFITS

This dish provides a generous serving of vegetables, with omega-3 fatty acids from the anchovies. Red bell peppers and tomatoes are excellent sources of carotenoids and vitamin C.

Per serving: 5g protein, 9g carbohydrate, 5g fat, 3g fiber, 95 calories/400 kJ

SIMPLE SALADS

A Salad and a slice of whole-grain, nut, or seed bread (see pages 226 and 227) can be the basis of a nutritionally complete lunch or supper, as long as you include some protein, such as poached or boiled eggs, cottage cheese, shrimp, smoked fish, cooked chicken or turkey. Try some of these suggestions:

- *Avocados, tomatoes, mozzarella cheese, and fresh basil, drizzled with extra-virgin olive oil and balsamic vinegar*
- *Beets, arugula, and walnuts, with walnut oil vinaigrette*
- *Fresh baby fava beans with cubes of mild Pecorino Romano cheese, drizzled with extra-virgin olive oil*
- *Belgian endive, walnuts, and Roquefort cheese, with walnut oil vinaigrette*
- *Greek salad of romaine lettuce, tomatoes, cucumber, green bell pepper, red onion, feta cheese, dried oregano, black olives, with extra-virgin olive oil and lemon juice dressing*
- *Shrimp and cubed canteloupe with cherry tomatoes, cucumber, and mixed lettuces, with olive oil vinaigrette*

Leeks with Cranberry Vinaigrette

Serve as a first course, or with cold turkey or lean pork for a complete meal.

SERVES 4

2 large or 3 medium leeks

20 fresh or frozen cranberries

2 tablespoons orange juice

1 tablespoon walnut oil

1 teaspoon good-quality
red wine vinegar

Salt and freshly ground
black pepper

TRIM the leeks, but don't discard too much of the green part; wash well, and slice in thin rounds. Steam or boil the leeks until they are soft but not mushy.

MEANWHILE, make the vinaigrette: Heat the cranberries and orange juice in a medium saucepan over low heat until the cranberries begin to soften. Remove from the heat, allow to cool, then put the mixture in a blender with the oil, vinegar, and salt and pepper to taste. Blend just enough to mix well but leaving visible bits of cranberry.

DRAIN the leeks thoroughly and, if necessary, pat dry on paper towels. While the leeks are still slightly warm, put them in a serving bowl, add the vinaigrette, and mix thoroughly. Serve at room temperature.

NUTRITIONAL BENEFITS

This light, fresh-tasting salad provides a serving of vegetables and is a delicious way to get the prebiotic benefits of leeks.

Per serving: 1g protein, 9g carbohydrate, 4g fat, 1g fiber, 65 calories/273 kJ

Carrot and Parsley Salad
with Pomegranate Vinaigrette

A vibrantly colorful winter first course, or an accompaniment to grilled fish

serves 4

1 pomegranate

1 tablespoon extra-virgin olive oil

1 clove garlic, crushed

Juice of ½ lemon

Salt and freshly ground black pepper

2¼ cups grated carrots

1 large bunch of parsley,

* leaves chopped*

Cut the pomegranate in half. Squeeze the juice from half the pomegranate, and remove the seeds from the other half.

In a lidded jar or other container, combine the pomegranate juice, oil, garlic, a good squeeze of lemon juice, and salt and pepper to taste. Shake well.

In a serving bowl, combine the carrots and parsley. Dress with the vinaigrette and mix well. Sprinkle the pomegranate seeds over the salad, and serve.

CARROT AND CRANBERRY SALAD

Replace the pomegranate juice with the juice of 1 additional lemon. Add 1 cup chopped fresh cranberries to the salad and a few walnuts if you like.

NUTRITIONAL BENEFITS

The combination of carrots and parsley makes a good serving of carotene-rich vegetables—you will get all the vitamin A you need for a day from this salad. It also provides more than a third of your daily vitamin C and plenty of vitamin K. Pomegranates contribute to your daily polyphenol intake.

Per serving: 1g protein, 14g carbohydrate, 4g fat, 2g fiber, 88 calories/370 kJ

Celeriac and Apple Salad

This salad makes a satisfying lunch, and is excellent with hot or cold chicken. If you are making it more than an hour in advance, toss the celeriac and apples in lemon juice before mixing to prevent them from turning brown.

serves 4

FOR THE DRESSING:

½ tablespoon white wine
   vinegar or cider vinegar
Juice of ½ lemon
1 teaspoon Dijon mustard
2 cloves garlic, crushed
Salt and freshly ground black pepper
1 tablespoon extra-virgin olive oil
⅔ cup low-fat plain yogurt

7 ounces celeriac (half
   a medium-size root),
   peeled and grated
2 apples, skin left on, coarsely
   chopped
1 small red onion, finely chopped
¾ cup chopped walnuts

First, Make the dressing: Whisk together the vinegar, lemon juice, mustard, garlic, and salt and pepper to taste, then whisk in the oil. Finally, whisk in the yogurt.

Combine the celeriac, apples, onion, and walnuts in a large bowl. Add the dressing, toss to coat the salad, and serve.

NUTRITIONAL BENEFITS

A generous serving of this salad contains small amounts of all the B-group vitamins, plus some vitamin C. The apples and walnuts provide procyanidins and other protective polyphenols. The walnuts make it rather high in fat, but very little of this fat is saturated.

Per serving: 6g protein, 22g carbohydrate, 17g fat, 4g fiber, 252 calories/1058 kJ

Persimmon, Smoked Chicken, and Avocado Salad

Smoked chicken and lots of greens will make this salad into a complete meal, but it's equally good without the chicken as a first course.

serves 4

FOR THE DRESSING:
3 tablespoons extra-virgin olive oil
1 tablespoon good-quality
    red wine vinegar
¼ teaspoon sugar
1 heaping teaspoon dry mustard
1 clove garlic, crushed

3 persimmons
2 small avocados
1 red onion, very finely chopped
10 ounces smoked chicken, chopped

FIRST, make the dressing: Combine all the dressing ingredients in a lidded jar or other container and shake well.

WASH the persimmons and remove the leaves and bases. Chop into bite-size pieces. Skin and pit the avocados and chop them into bite-size pieces. Combine the persimmons, avocados, and onion in a serving bowl, pour over the dressing, and toss to mix. Add the smoked chicken and serve.

NUTRITIONAL BENEFITS

This salad makes for an unusual way to take advantage of the polyphenols in persimmons. Avocados are a good source of healthy monounsaturated fats and vitamin E. The salad also provides a good mix of other vitamins and minerals.

Per serving: 26g protein, 15g carbohydrate, 21g fat, 5g fiber, 343 calories/1436 kJ

Lentil, Spinach, and Feta Cheese Salad

This is a substantial salad that can be served as a main meal. To reduce the fat content, use low-fat feta cheese and sun-dried tomatoes that are not packed in oil.

SERVES 2

¾ cup green lentils

4 ounces fresh baby spinach

1 small red onion, finely chopped

1 ounce sun-dried tomatoes, chopped

2 ounces feta cheese, diced

¼ cup roughly chopped walnuts

FOR THE DRESSING:

½ teaspoon Dijon mustard

1 clove garlic, crushed

Freshly ground black pepper

2 tablespoons extra-virgin olive oil

½ tablespoons balsamic vinegar

WASH the lentils thoroughly, then put them in a saucepan with 1¼ cups water, bring to a boil, then reduce the heat and simmer until the water has been absorbed and the lentils are tender, 15 to 20 minutes.

MEANWHILE, make the dressing: Whisk together the mustard, garlic, and pepper to taste, then whisk in the oil and vinegar. Taste and adjust the seasoning—you may not need to add salt.

PUT the hot lentils in a medium bowl, add the dressing, and mix well. Add the spinach and set aside to cool.

MIX in the red onion, sun-dried tomatoes, feta, and walnuts. Serve on a bed of lettuce, arugula, watercress, or mixed greens.

NUTRITIONAL BENEFITS

This salad is a good source of vegetable protein, with a little cheese to enhance the flavor. One serving has a day's supply of folate, along with plenty of other B-group vitamins. It's also packed with carotenoids, vitamins C, E, and K, plus iron, calcium, phosphorus, and zinc.

Per serving: 23g protein, 4g carbohydrate, 30g fat, 16g fiber, 533 calories/2238 kJ

Turkey, Rice, and Bean Salad

This main course salad is a lovely mixture of colors, flavors, and textures.

serves 4

1 cup adzuki beans or black
  beans, soaked overnight

½ cup brown rice

2 tablespoons extra-virgin olive oil

2 teaspoons white wine vinegar

½ teaspoon Dijon mustard

Salt and freshly ground black pepper

1 large green bell pepper, chopped

½ cucumber, chopped

1 red onion, finely chopped

½ cup dried cranberries

½ cup roughly chopped walnuts

7 ounces cooked turkey, chicken,
  or lean ham, chopped

Drain the soaked beans, place in a saucepan, cover with cold water—do not add salt—and bring to a boil for 10 minutes. Reduce the heat and simmer for 30 to 50 minutes, until tender. Drain well.

Cook the rice in a saucepan of lightly salted boiling water for 25 to 35 minutes, or until tender. Drain and rinse under cold running water.

Whisk together the oil, vinegar, mustard, and salt and pepper to taste. Stir the dressing into the beans while they are still warm.

When the mixture has cooled, stir in the remaining ingredients. Serve on a bed of lettuce leaves.

NUTRITIONAL BENEFITS

The combination of beans, cranberries, and walnuts puts some protective polyphenols on your plate. Bell pepper, cucumber, and red onion give you a generous serving of vegetables. The salad is a good source of vitamin C, folate, and B-group vitamins, along with selenium, zinc, and iron.

Per serving: 28g protein, 58g carbohydrate, 19g fat, 12g fiber, 503 calories/2112 kJ

Chicken, Orange, and Fennel Salad

A great way to use leftover roast chicken—or try it with duck if you like. As a variation, you could use baby spinach leaves or arugula instead of the watercress, or a mixture of the three if you prefer.

SERVES 4

3 large oranges
1 fennel bulb
2 tablespoons extra-virgin olive oil
Dash of soy sauce (preferably tamari)
Juice of 1 lemon
Salt and freshly ground black pepper

1 bunch (about 7 ounces)
watercress
7 ounces cooked chicken, cut
into bite-size pieces
⅛ cup roughly chopped
walnuts

HOLDING the oranges over a bowl to catch the juice, peel them with a sharp knife, making sure you remove all the white pith. Cut the oranges into segments, discarding the pits.

TRIM any tough or discolored parts from the fennel, then cut into thin slices.

IN a medium bowl, whisk together the oil, soy sauce, and reserved orange juice, then whisk in the lemon juice and salt and pepper to taste.

COMBINE the watercress, fennel, orange segments, and chicken, and place on a plate. Sprinkle the walnuts on top and drizzle with the dressing.

NUTRITIONAL BENEFITS

This salad is a fantastic source of vitamins A, C, and K, and also provides B-group vitamins, particularly niacin and B_6, plus a range of minerals, including calcium and magnesium.

Per serving: 20g protein, 23g carbohydrate, 15g fat, 6g fiber, 298 calories/1251 kJ

Salade Niçoise

Mediterranean summer on a plate, this salad is equally good with fresh or canned tuna. The corn is not strictly authentic, but it adds color; you could use diced red or yellow bell pepper instead.

serves 4

14 ounces small new potatoes

5 ounces small green beans

1 small onion, very finely chopped

2 tablespoons extra-virgin olive oil

1 tablespoon good-quality
    red wine vinegar

Salt and freshly ground black pepper

7 ounces canned tuna in water,
    drained and flaked, or 7 ounces
    fresh tuna, cut into 4- by
    ½-inch-thick slices

2 heads romaine lettuce,
    chopped

1½ cups boiled or
    canned corn kernels

4 tomatoes, quartered

4 hard-boiled eggs, quartered
    lengthwise

16 small black olives

2 ounces anchovies
    (optional)

In a large saucepan of lightly salted water, boil the potatoes in their skins until just tender, about 20 minutes. Drain and cut the potatoes in half. In another saucepan, boil the green beans until just tender, about 10 minutes. Drain and refresh quickly under cold running water. Drain well. Combine the potatoes, green beans, and onion in a large bowl.

In a medium bowl, whisk together the oil, vinegar, and salt and pepper to taste and toss with the potatoes, beans, and onion.

If you are using fresh tuna, cook it very quickly in a hot nonstick skillet or grill pan—do not overcook or it will be tasteless.

Divide the lettuce among 4 serving plates. Top with the potato and bean salad, followed by the corn, and then the tuna. Arrange the tomatoes, eggs, and olives around the plates, along with the anchovies, if using, and serve at once.

ITALIAN-STYLE MIXED GREENS

This dish is a tasty and versatile accompaniment to just about any main course. It traditionally includes wild greens, such as dandelions, but you can use whatever green vegetables are in season: cabbage, kale, collard greens, watercress, arugula, romaine lettuce, spinach, Swiss chard, fennel, zucchini, green beans, leeks, or scallions.

SERVES 4

7 ounces savoy cabbage or kale,
  tough stems removed
2 large or 3 medium leeks
1 fennel bulb
2 tablespoons extra-virgin olive oil
2 to 3 cloves garlic, sliced

¼ teaspoon crushed dried
  chiles (red chile flakes)
Up to 1 cup vegetable stock
Salt and freshly ground
  black pepper
1 lemon, halved

WASH and prepare the vegetables: Shred or chop the cabbage and slice the leeks and fennel into bite-size pieces.

HEAT the oil in a large saucepan over low heat. Add the garlic and cook for 30 seconds, until fragrant. Add the vegetables and stir well to coat in the garlicky oil.

ADD the chiles and a little stock—a few tablespoons will be enough to cook leafy vegetables; firmer vegetables such as fennel will need more. Cover and simmer until the vegetables are tender, up to 20 minutes. Season with salt and pepper to taste and squeeze the lemon juice over top. Serve hot.

LEFTOVERS will make a good soup the next day: Blend to a purée, then thin down with vegetable stock.

NUTRITIONAL BENEFITS

This dish makes it easy to get two servings of vegetables and plenty of vitamin C with your lunch or dinner. Depending on the vegetables you choose, it can also be a good source of carotenoids, folate, or other nutrients. The fat is mainly healthy monounsaturated fat from the olive oil.

Per serving: 2g protein, 12g carbohydrate, 7g fat, 4g fiber, 110 calories/462 kJ

Bean and Tomato Casserole

Dried beans have a better flavor and texture than canned ones—and they're about a quarter of the price. Serve as a vegetarian lunch or to accompany grilled lean lamb or chicken. This recipe can be made in double quantities— it freezes well.

serves 4

⅛ cup dried great Northern
   or white beans
¼ cup dried soybeans
¼ cup dried pinto or
   cranberry beans
1 tablespoon extra-virgin olive oil
1 clove garlic, crushed

1 red onion, finely chopped
1 green bell pepper, chopped
One 14-ounce can chopped
   tomatoes
Salt and freshly ground black
   pepper
2 tablespoons chopped fresh basil

SOAK the beans overnight in cold water. Drain the beans and rinse well.

HEAT the oil in a large, heavy-bottomed saucepan over low heat. Add the garlic and onion and cook for for 3 minutes, or until softened. Add the beans and cook for an additional 3 minutes, stirring occasionally. Pour over enough boiling water to cover the beans, and boil for 10 minutes, then reduce the heat and simmer until tender, about 1 hour.

VERSATILE BEAN PURÉE

Protein-packed bean or pea purées can be served as a dip or as an accompaniment to fish and grilled meats. Season the purées with salt and pepper to taste.

- *Cook frozen fava beans and peas in boiling water, then blend with 2 teaspoons tahini (sesame seed paste), 1 to 2 cloves garlic, the juice of ½ lemon, and a little of the pea cooking water to desired consistency.*
- *Blend cooked or canned lima beans, 3 cloves garlic, and a little olive oil.*
- *Cook frozen peas in boiling water, then run under cold water to set the green color. Blend with one tablespoon of chopped fresh mint and 1 to 2 tablespoons plain yogurt.*

ADD the bell pepper and tomatoes, season lightly with salt and pepper, and continue cooking until reduced to a thick consistency. Add the chopped basil just before serving.

NUTRITIONAL BENEFITS

Mixed beans provide complete protein, and this dish is the equivalent of two servings of vegetables. And there's plenty of vitamin C, plus folate, iron, and magnesium.

Per serving: 11g protein, 26g carbohydrate, 6g fat, 10g fiber, 193 calories/810kJ

WALNUT PILAF

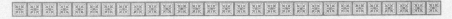

For a colorful Middle Eastern touch—and extra polyphenols—stir in some fresh pomegranate seeds just before serving. Serve as an accompaniment to roast chicken or turkey, or with a green salad for lunch.

*3½ cups well-flavored chicken
or vegetable stock*

1 teaspoon extra-virgin olive oil

1 onion, finely chopped

1 clove garlic, finely chopped

1 cup long-grain brown rice

1 teaspoon ground cinnamon

*4 ready-to-eat dried apricots,
cut into slivers*

½ cup roughly chopped walnuts

*1 large bunch of parsley,
leaves chopped*

*Salt and freshly ground
black pepper*

BRING the stock to a boil in a large saucepan. Meanwhile, heat the oil in a large saucepan over low heat. Add the onion and garlic and cook until softened, about 5 minutes. Add the rice and cinnamon and stir to mix well. Add the boiling stock, cover with a lid, then reduce the heat and simmer for 20 to 25 minutes, until the rice is tender.

STIR in the apricots, walnuts, and parsley, and heat through for a few minutes. Season with salt and pepper to taste and serve hot.

VARIATIONS

⬤ Try using pine nuts instead of the walnuts; toast them lightly before adding them to the pilaf.

⬤ Use the mixture to fill 4 large red bell peppers. First cut the peppers in half lengthwise and seed them, then brush lightly all over with olive oil. Place the peppers in a roasting pan and fill with the pilaf. Bake in a preheated oven at 400°F for about 1 hour.

NUTRITIONAL BENEFITS

Using lots of parsley boosts the vitamin and mineral content of this pilaf; the pilaf also contains protective polyphenols from the walnuts and cinnamon.

Per serving: 5g protein, 27g carbohydrate, 10g fat, 4g fiber, 209 calories/876 kJ

Tabbouleh

This fresh-tasting herb, tomato, and bulgur wheat salad makes a great lunch dish. It's also a good accompaniment to barbecued chicken, meat, or fish. Check whether the bulgur wheat you buy can be prepared simply by soaking or if it needs to be cooked.

serves 4

1 ¼ cups bulgur wheat

4 ripe tomatoes

1 small red onion, finely chopped

1 clove garlic, finely
    chopped (optional)

1 tablespoon extra-virgin olive oil

Grated zest and juice of 1 lemon

1 bunch of parsley, leaves chopped

1 bunch of mint, leaves chopped

1 bunch of cilantro, leaves chopped

Salt and freshly ground
    black pepper

Put the bulgur in a large bowl and pour over enough boiling water to cover by ½ inch. Cover and leave to soak for 10 minutes, then fluff up with a fork. Meanwhile, slice the tomatoes in half and scoop out most of the seeds; cut the flesh into small dice.

Add the onion, garlic, oil, lemon zest and juice, and herbs to the bulgur wheat and stir well. Season with salt and pepper to taste, then gently stir in the tomatoes.

The tabbouleh can be stored, covered, in the refrigerator for up to 3 days.

NUTRITIONAL BENEFITS

This is a tasty change from rice or potatoes, with a relatively low glycemic load. It contains more than half your daily vitamin C.

Per serving: 7g protein, 42g carbohydrate, 4g fat, 10g fiber, 218 calories/915 kJ

Collard Green Loaf with Spicy Tomato Sauce

This vegetarian main course could also be served as a first course for six to eight people.

SERVES 4

1½ pounds collard greens
1 tablespoon extra-virgin olive oil
1 onion, finely chopped
2 cloves garlic, chopped
¾ cup whole-wheat bread crumbs
2 large eggs, beaten
¼ teaspoon freshly grated nutmeg
Salt and freshly ground black pepper
3 hard-boiled eggs, shelled

TOMATO SAUCE

1 teaspoon extra-virgin olive oil
2 cloves garlic, minced
3 small dried chiles
One 14-ounce can
   chopped tomatoes

PREHEAT the oven to 350°F. Oil a small loaf pan.

WASH the greens. Set aside 4 to 6 large outer leaves to line the pan; cut out their central stems. Trim off any tough stems and chop the rest of the greens. Put them in the basket of a steamer and place the reserved whole leaves on top. Cover and steam for about 3 minutes, then remove the whole leaves, which should be slightly wilted; use them to line the pan. Continue steaming the rest of the greens for another 10 minutes, or until quite tender, then remove from the heat and blend them in a food processor.

HEAT the oil in a small saucepan over low heat. Add the onion and garlic and cook until softened, about 5 minutes. In a large bowl, combine the bread crumbs, the blended greens, beaten eggs, onion, garlic, nutmeg, and salt and pepper to taste. Put about half the mixture in the lined pan. Press the hard-boiled eggs lengthwise down the middle of the pan and cover them with the rest of the mixture. Press gently to flatten, and fold over any protruding bits of leaf. Cover with foil and place in a deep roasting pan; add boiling water to come halfway up the sides of the loaf pan. Cook for 40 minutes, or until firm to the touch.

MEANWHILE, make the sauce: Heat the oil in a medium saucepan over medium heat. Add the garlic and chiles and cook until the garlic is fragrant, about 30 seconds. Add the tomatoes and cook until the sauce is thick, about 15 to 20 minutes. Remove the chiles.

LEAVE the loaf to cool slightly, then invert it onto a plate. Slice and serve with the tomato sauce. The loaf can be served at any temperature but is best at room temperature.

NUTRITIONAL BENEFITS

Collard greens—a type of cabbage—are an excellent source of carotenoids, vitamin C, and folate. This dish also gives you plenty of other vitamins and minerals—nearly a third of your calcium and nearly half your iron.

Per serving: 15g protein, 31g carbohydrate, 12g fat, 9g fiber, 282 calories/1184 kJ

Nut Roast

Any two types of nuts will work for this roast. You can try cashews, or if you picked pistachio nuts, use a maximum of half a cup (about 2 ounces) and don't chop them—stir the nuts whole into the mixture. Instead of cheddar cheese, you can try Monterey Jack, Parmesan, or Pecorino Romano. The rice can be cooked a day ahead and stored, covered, in the refrigerator. Any leftovers will be great served cold the next day.

SERVES 6 TO 8

½ cup brown rice

1 tablespoon extra-virgin olive oil

2 onions, finely chopped

2 carrots, grated

1 clove garlic, crushed

7 ounces mushrooms, finely chopped

1½ cups fresh whole-wheat
   bread crumbs

⅓ cup finely chopped Brazil nuts

½ cup finely chopped walnuts

½ cup finely chopped almonds

¼ cup shredded Cheddar cheese

2 large eggs, beaten

1 tablespoon chopped fresh
   oregano or basil

2 tablespoons chopped fresh parsley

Salt and freshly ground
   black pepper

Cook the rice in a saucepan of lightly salted boiling water for 25 to 30 minutes, or until tender. Drain and rinse under cold running water.

Preheat the oven to 375°F. Oil a large loaf pan.

Heat the oil in a large saucepan over low heat. Add the onions, carrots, and garlic and cook for 5 minutes, or until softened. Add the mushrooms and cook, stirring often, until tender, approximately 10 minutes. Remove from the heat and stir in the bread crumbs, cooked rice, nuts, cheese, eggs, and herbs. Season with salt and pepper to taste. Spoon into the loaf pan and bake for about 1 hour, or until firm to the touch and lightly browned on top. Serve hot or cold with tomato sauce (see page 253) and a generous helping of green vegetables or salad.

NUTRITIONAL BENEFITS

Served with broccoli, this is a nutritious—if somewhat high-fat—meal. Nuts are high in healthy fats and also are a good source of protein (especially in combination with whole-wheat bread, brown rice, and cheese), along with a whole range of vitamins, minerals, and trace elements.

Per serving (with 1 cup cooked broccoli): 14g protein, 32g carbohydrate, 22g fat, 9g fiber, 359 calories/1508 kJ

Spaghetti with Walnut and Eggplant Sauce

Eggplants are sometimes described as the poor man's meat; they give this dish a rich, meaty taste.

serves 4

2 large or 3 medium eggplants
⅔ cup coarsely chopped walnuts
1 clove garlic
2 tablespoons extra-virgin olive oil
Salt and freshly ground
   black pepper

10 ounces whole-wheat spaghetti
2 ounces Parmesan cheese,
   finely grated
1 large bunch of parsley,
   leaves chopped

Preheat the oven to 375°F. Prick the eggplants in several places with a fork, put them in a lightly oiled roasting pan, and bake for 20 to 30 minutes, or until soft.

When the eggplants are cool enough to handle, peel off the skins and put the flesh in a blender with the walnuts and garlic. Blend, adding 1 tablespoon oil to give a creamy consistency. Add salt and pepper to taste. Put in a saucepan with the remaining oil and warm the sauce in a saucepan.

Cook the spaghetti in a pot of lightly salted boiling water until al dente. Drain. Add the pasta to the sauce, remove from the heat, and mix well. Add the Parmesan and mix again. Serve immediately, sprinkled with the parsley, and a generous helping of salad alongside.

NUTRITIONAL BENEFITS

A good source of a whole range of vitamins and minerals, this dish provides a third of your daily vitamin C and iron, along with vitamins A, E, K, and B-group vitamins. It is also a good source of calcium, phosphorus, magnesium, selenium, and zinc. The walnuts provide protective polyphenols.

Per serving: 21g protein, 76g carbohydrate, 21g fat, 11g fiber, 534 calories/2243 kJ

Spaghetti with Tomato and Anchovy Sauce

A simple Mediterranean-style supper. You could add some black olives, if you like or, for a spicier sauce, add ¹/4 teaspoon crushed dried chiles along with the garlic. Serve with a large green or mixed salad.

SERVES 2

1 tablespoon extra-virgin olive oil
3 cloves garlic, crushed
2 ounces canned anchovy
    fillets, snipped
1 pound fresh ripe tomatoes, skinned,
    seeded, and roughly chopped,

or one 14-ounce can
    chopped tomatoes
Freshly ground black pepper
5 ounces whole-wheat spaghetti
2 tablespoon roughly chopped
    fresh basil

Heat the oil in a medium saucepan over low heat. Add the garlic and anchovies and cook for 2 to 3 minutes, until softened. Add the tomatoes and pepper to taste and simmer for about 30 minutes, or until thickened.

Cook the spaghetti in a pot of lightly salted boiling water until al dente, then drain. Add the spaghetti to the sauce, along with the basil. Remove from the heat and mix well. Serve immediately.

NUTRITIONAL BENEFITS

Tomatoes are an excellent source of the carotenoid lycopene—and they count as one serving of vegetables. This dish is also a good source of a surprisingly wide range of vitamins and minerals.

Per serving: 19g protein, 66g carbohydrate, 10g fat, 2g fiber, 410 calories/1722 kJ

Salmon with Watercress-Tofu Sauce

The watercress makes for a bright green, peppery-tasting sauce. For a gentler flavor the watercress can be blanched for 10 seconds in boiling water and drained thoroughly before blending it with the tofu. Use organic or wild salmon.

serves 2

Two 5-ounce salmon fillets
2 tablespoons lemon juice
  or white wine
1 bunch of watercress, large
  stalks removed
4 ounces silken tofu

Juice of ½ lemon
1 clove garlic, crushed
Salt and freshly ground
  black pepper
2 tablespoons capers, drained

Preheat the oven to 375°F. Place each salmon fillet on a piece of aluminum foil, drizzle with the the lemon juice, then fold the foil up over the salmon parcels to seal. Bake for about 15 to 20 minutes, or until the salmon is cooked through.

MEANWHILE, make the watercress-tofu sauce: Place the watercress, tofu, lemon juice, garlic, and salt and pepper to taste in a food processor and blend until smooth. Stir in the capers.

SERVE the salmon hot with the cold watercress sauce, accompanied by baked tomatoes, braised endive, and new potatoes boiled in their skins.

NUTRITIONAL BENEFITS

High in healthy omega-3 fats, this dish is also a good source of beta-carotene, lutein, and zeaxanthin, plus vitamins C, K, and the whole B group. It makes a useful contribution to your daily calcium, phosphorus, iron, and zinc intakes.

Per serving: 42g protein, 6g carbohydrate, 14g fat, 1g fiber, 320 calories/1344 kJ

SALMON WITH RYE AND KIDNEY BEANS

All you need to accompany this dish is some lemony mayonnaise—or a mixture of half mayonnaise and half yogurt—and a salad or steamed green vegetables. You can find rye grains in health food stores; they're very filling, so you won't need a lot. Be sure to use organic or wild salmon.

SERVES 4

¾ cup whole rye

One 10-ounce fillet of salmon

1¼ cups cooked or canned
   red kidney beans

1 large bunch of parsley,
   leaves chopped

Salt and freshly ground
   black pepper

BOIL the rye in a large pot of water for about 45 minutes, or until tender but still al dente. Drain.

PREHEAT the oven to 375°F. Put the salmon in a baking dish, add a little water, cover the dish with foil, and poach the salmon in the oven for about 15 minutes; it should be flaky but still moist. Flake the salmon using a kitchen fork.

PLACE the rye, kidney beans, and gently flaked salmon in a warmed serving dish, sprinkle with the parsley, season with salt and pepper to taste, and mix well. Serve at room temperature.

NUTRITIONAL BENEFITS

Salmon is a source of healthy omega-3 fatty acids. Kidney beans and rye provide plant protein to complement the protein in the salmon. Parsley contains plenty of vitamin C, folate, and carotene, so use as much as you like.

Per serving: 30g protein, 39g carbohydrate, 7g fat, 10g fiber, 338 calories/1420 kJ

Monkfish Kebabs with Pomegranate Salsa

Monkfish is the perfect fish for kebabs, as it doesn't fall apart when cooked.

SERVES 4

2 pomegranates

1 pound monkfish, skinned, filleted, and cut into cubes

About 48 plum or cherry tomatoes

1 bunch of flat-leaf parsley, leaves finely chopped

2 cloves garlic, crushed

1 or 2 small red chiles, very finely chopped

1 to 2 tablespoons extra-virgin olive oil

Salt and freshly ground black pepper

ABOUT an hour before you plan cook the kebabs, juice one of the pomegranates on a lemon squeezer and marinate the monkfish in the juice. (You can do this up to 24 hours ahead—cover the bowl and keep it refrigerated, turning the fish occasionally.)

ASSEMBLE the kebabs: Thread 8 skewers with alternating pieces of monkfish (which will now be a pretty shade of pale pink) and tomatoes. Broil the kebabs (or grill them outdoors), turning 2 or 3 times; they will need a total of about 15 minutes.

WHILE the kebabs are cooking, prepare the salsa. Cut the remaining pomegranate in half and scoop out the seeds into a serving bowl, removing any bits of pith. Don't worry if this creates quite a bit of juice—it's all part of the plan. Add the parsley, garlic, chopped chiles, and enough olive oil to reach your desired consistency. Mix well and season with salt and pepper to taste.

SERVE with brown rice, couscous, tabbouleh (see page 252), or a bean or pea purée (see page 250).

NUTRITIONAL BENEFITS

Pomegranates are full of protective polyphenols—an added bonus in this already healthful recipe.

Per serving: 25g protein, 21g carbohydrate, 7g fat, 2g fiber, 237 calories/995 kJ

Seared Tuna with Bean and Red Bell Pepper Salad

You can use any type of beans for this simple supper—I chose white beans to contrast with the red pepper.

SERVES 2

BEAN AND RED BELL PEPPER
SALAD
2 tablespoons extra-virgin olive oil
*2 teaspoons good-quality
    red wine vinegar*
1 teaspoon Dijon mustard
1 clove garlic, crushed
*Salt and freshly ground
    black pepper*

One 14-ounce can white beans, drained
1 large red onion, finely chopped
*1 head romaine lettuce,
roughly chopped*

Two 3.5-ounce fresh tuna steaks
3.5 ounces extra-virgin olive oil

FIRST, make the salad: Whisk together the oil, vinegar, mustard, garlic, and salt and pepper to taste. Heat the beans to warm through, then mix with the dressing and leave to cool. When cooled, stir in the bell pepper and onion. Toss with the lettuce.

HEAT a ridged grill pan or heavy nonstick pan over medium-high heat until hot. Brush the tuna with olive oil to coat lightly but evenly. Sear the tuna for no more than 2 minutes each side; it should still be pink in the middle and if overcooked will be tough and tasteless. Serve immediately with the bean salad.

NUTRITIONAL BENEFITS

There's plenty of healthy omega-3 fatty acids and fiber in this dish—and it's a really good source of most vitamins and minerals.

Per serving: 43g protein, 42g carbohydrate, 21g fat, 12g fiber, 521 calories/2188 kJ

SHRIMP AND PEANUT STIR-FRY

This dish is colorful, fragrant, and quick to cook—make sure all the ingredients are prepared and ready to throw into the wok. You can use precooked shrimp, but uncooked shrimp will have a better flavor.

serves 2

1 tablespoon extra-virgin olive oil

1 large onion, chopped

2 cloves garlic, chopped

1 or 2 fresh green chiles, seeded and chopped

1 red bell pepper, sliced

1 green bell pepper, sliced

4 ounces mushrooms, sliced

5 ounces peeled and deveined medium or large shrimp

⅛ cup frozen peas

⅛ cup shelled peanuts

1 tablespoon peanut butter

½ tablespoon soy sauce

Freshly ground black pepper

HEAT the oil in a wok or large nonstick saucepan over medium-high heat. Add the onion, garlic, chiles, bell peppers, and mushrooms and stir-fry until tender, about 5 minutes.

ADD the shrimp, peas, and peanuts and stir-fry for an additional 3 to 4 minutes, or until the shrimp is just cooked through. Add the peanut butter, soy sauce, and pepper to taste and stir to dissolve the peanut butter. Add 1 or 2 tablespoons of water if the stir-fry seems too dry. Serve immediately over brown rice.

NUTRITIONAL BENEFITS

Served with brown rice, this stir-fry includes 2 servings of vegetables and provides plenty of protein from a variety of sources. It is also packed with vitamins C, E, A, and the B group, and has about a third of your daily requirements for magnesium, iron, and zinc.

Per serving (with ½ cup rice): 33g protein, 52g carbohydrate, 26g fat, 11g fiber, 543 calories/2280 kJ

Broiled Mackerel with Beet and Cranberry Salad

The deep red warm salad makes for a great contrast to the intense flavor of the mackerel.

serves 4

*One 14-ounce can mixed
  beans, drained*
Scant 1 cup dried cranberries
*2 tablespoons extra-virgin
  olive oil*
Juice of 1 lemon
5 ounces cooked beets, diced

1 bunch of scallions, chopped
*1 large bunch of flat-leaf
  parsley, leaves chopped*
*Salt and freshly ground
  black pepper*
*Four 5-ounce fresh mackerel
  or bluefish fillets*

In a small saucepan, heat the beans, cranberries, and olive oil gently to warm through, then mix in the lemon juice, beets, scallions, parsley, and salt and pepper to taste.

Cook the fish fillets under the broiler or on the barbecue for about 2 minutes on each side, or until cooked through. Serve hot, with the beet and cranberry salad and new potatoes boiled in their skins.

NUTRITIONAL BENEFITS

It's often said that fish is good for the brain, and this recipe is packed with nearly a week's supply of vitamin B_{12}, which recently has been linked with cognitive function (see page 204). It's also high in omega-3 fatty acids, and it contains protective polyphenols from the cranberries.

Per serving: 45g protein, 53g carbohydrate, 31g fat, 13g fiber, 667 calories/2801 kJ

Baked Fish with Tomatoes and Olives

A simple, aromatic midweek supper with all the flavors of the Mediterranean.

SERVES 2

*1 tablespoon extra-virgin
  olive oil*

1 onion, finely chopped

1 clove garlic, crushed

*1 pound fresh ripe tomatoes,
  skinned, seeded, and roughly
  chopped, or one 14-ounce can
  chopped tomatoes*

Salt and freshly ground black pepper

*2 to 3 tablespoons roughly
  chopped fresh basil*

*2 to 3 tablespoons chopped fresh
  flat-leaf parsley*

2 5-ounce whitefish fillets

Juice of ½ lemon

10 to 12 black olives

HEAT the oil in a large saucepan over low heat. Add the onion and garlic and cook for 5 minutes, until softened. Add the tomatoes, season with a little salt and pepper, and simmer, uncovered, for 30 minutes, or until thickened. Stir in the basil and parsley.

MEANWHILE, preheat the oven to 375°F. Put the fish in a shallow baking dish, season with pepper to taste and the lemon juice, then spoon the sauce over the fish and top with the olives. Cover and bake for 20 to 25 minutes, or until the fish is cooked through. Serve with mixed brown and wild rice and a green salad.

Tomatoes and herbs provide a generous serving of vegetables in this dish, adding vitamins A and C to the B vitamins from the fish. A range of other vitamins and minerals complete the picture.

Per serving: 37g protein, 19g carbohydrate, 9g fat, 4g fiber, 301 calories/1264 kJ

Squid and Fennel Stew with Barley

An all-in-one pot dinner inspired by Mediterranean fish stews.

serves 4

¾ cup pearl barley

2 tablespoons extra-virgin
   olive oil

3 cloves garlic, chopped

2 small dried chiles

Handful of fresh parsley,
   chopped

14 ounces squid, cleaned and
   cut into rings

Good pinch of saffron, infused
   in a little boiling water

9 ounces cherry tomatoes

2 large fennel bulbs,
   roughly chopped

10 to 12 whole black
   peppercorns
   (optional)

Salt

Cook the barley in a large pot of boiling water for about 30 minutes, or until tender. Drain.

Warm the oil in a cast-iron pot over low heat. Add the garlic and chiles and cook for 2 minutes, or until softened. Add the parsley, stir, and then add the squid. Cook over low heat for about 5 minutes, then add the saffron. Remove the chiles (unless you don't mind eating them—they will be harder to remove once you have added the tomatoes!). Add the tomatoes, fennel, barley, and peppercorns, if using. Mix well, reduce the heat to a very low, and cook for about 1½ hours, until fennel is tender. Stir and check from time to time, adding a little water if necessary to prevent sticking. Season with salt to taste, and serve with a green salad.

Barley has a medium-low glycemic load and plenty of dietary fiber, making this a satisfying supper. It's got plenty of vitamins and minerals—including 75 percent of your daily vitamin C—and a good ratio of omega-3 to omega-6 fatty acids.

Per serving: 22g protein, 45g carbohydrate, 9g fat, 11g fiber, 340 calories/1428 kJ

Spicy Chicken Mole

My version of a Mexican dish that uses unsweetened chocolate as a spice. The chocolate is not particularly noticeable in the finished dish, but it lends a satisfying richness and body as well as, of course, providing important polyphenols. In Mexico this dish is likely to be made with turkey, rabbit, or game—why not try it with venison?

serves 4

1 tablespoon extra-virgin olive oil

1 large onion, chopped

2 cloves garlic, chopped

2 to 3 small dried chiles, chopped

1 large red bell pepper, sliced

7 ounces butternut squash, peeled and cubed

9 ounces skinless chicken breasts, cubed

One 14-ounce can chopped tomatoes

1 cup cooked or canned red kidney beans

⅓ cup shelled peanuts

5 tablespoons unsweetened cocoa powder, sifted

Juice of 2 limes

2 tablespoons peanut butter

Salt and freshly ground black pepper

PREHEAT the oven to 300°F.

WARM the oil in a flameproof casserole over low heat. Add the onion, garlic, and chiles and cook until softened, about 5 minutes. Add the bell pepper, squash, and chicken and cook, stirring, until the chicken changes color all over. Add the tomatoes, kidney beans, and peanuts; mix well, then cover the casserole and transfer to the oven to cook until the squash is tender, about 1 hour. Alternatively, simmer on top of the stove for 20 to 30 minutes.

Mix the cocoa powder and lime juice to make a paste. Add to the casserole along with the peanut butter. Taste and season with salt and pepper to taste. Heat through for a few minutes. This dish is very rich, so it's best served with plain brown rice or quinoa, a tasty alternative that goes well with this dish, and a simple salad.

NUTRITIONAL BENEFITS

Red bell peppers, squash, and tomatoes provide one of your daily helpings of vegetables, and are rich sources of carotenoids (used in the body to make vitamin A). Red bell peppers and limes provide vitamin C. Red kidney beans and peanuts are healthy plant protein sources that complement the chicken. Cocoa polyphenols confer many of the same benefits as red wine.

Per serving: 34g protein, 48g carbohydrate, 18g fat, 12g fiber, 457 calories/1919 kJ

Basque Chicken

A satisfying and colorful one-pot meal.

SERVES 2

1 tablespoon extra-virgin olive oil

2 chicken legs

1 large onion, quartered

3 bell peppers (any color),
   cut into thick slices

2 cloves garlic, chopped

1 ounce sun-dried tomatoes, chopped

1¾ ounces chorizo
   sausage, chopped

½ cup brown rice

1 cup chicken stock

⅔ cup dry white wine

1 tablespoon tomato purée

1 tablespoon dried
   mixed herbs

1 teaspoon paprika

10 to 12 black olives

Preheat the oven to 350°F.

Heat half the oil in a flameproof casserole, over medium heat. Brown the chicken legs all over. Remove the chicken to a plate. Add the remaining oil, the onion, and bell peppers and cook for 5 to 10 minutes, until they begin to soften. Add the garlic, sun-dried tomatoes, and chorizo, then stir in the rice. Add the stock, wine, tomato purée, herbs, paprika, and olives. Bring to a simmer. Put the chicken on top, then cover the casserole, transfer to the oven and cook for 1 hour, or until the chicken is cooked through. Alternatively, simmer on top of the stove for 30 to 40 minutes, until the chicken is cooked through. Serve hot.

NUTRITIONAL BENEFITS

The bell peppers have abundant vitamin C and carotenoids, and the onion provides pre-biotics. This dish is also a good source of vitamins E, K, and the B group and gives you a third of your daily iron, magnesium, zinc, and selenium.

Per serving: 39g protein, 49g carbohydrate, 27g fat, 10g fiber, 611 calories/2566 kJ

Faisanjin (Chicken with Pomegranates and Walnuts)

A food processor makes it quick and easy to chop the herbs and walnuts. A juicer helps with the pomegranates: Scoop out the seeds and pith, and pass through the juicer, and you don't have to worry about separating the pith from the seeds.

serves 4

1 tablespoon extra-virgin
   olive oil
10 ounces skinless chicken breasts,
   cut into bite-size chunks
1 large onion, sliced
2 cloves garlic, crushed

2 tablespoon tomato purée
One 14-ounce can
   chopped tomatoes
1 bunch flat-leaf parsley,
   leaves finely chopped

1 bunch mint, leaves	*Juice of 1 lime*
finely chopped	*1 cup finely chopped walnuts*
1 bunch cilantro, leaves	*Salt and freshly ground*
finely chopped	*black pepper*
Juice of 3 large or 4 small pome-	
granates (approximately 1¼ cups)	

WARM the oil in a large skillet over medium heat. Add the chicken, onion, and garlic and cook, stirring from time to time, until the onion is soft and the chicken is evenly browned, 10 to 15 minutes. Add the tomato purée and chopped tomatoes and simmer for 10 to 15 minutes, until the chicken is cooked through.

ADD the chopped herbs, and pomegranate and lime juices, and bring back to a simmer. Stir in the walnuts, season with salt and pepper to taste, and heat through. The shorter the reheating time, the more protective polyphenols will remain in the pomegranate juice and walnuts.

SERVE with brown rice and Middle Eastern vegetables (recipe follows).

MIDDLE EASTERN–STYLE VEGETABLES

HEAT 1 tablespoon olive oil in a large nonstick saucepan. Add 6 cubed baby eggplants, 2 small quartered red onions, 7 ounces green beans cut into 1½-inch lengths, and the juice of 2 limes. Cover the pan and cook over medium-high heat, stirring occasionally, until the beans and onion are just tender. Season to taste with salt and pepper and stir in a large handful of fresh herbs—parsley, mint, or cilantro.

NUTRITIONAL BENEFITS

With the suggested accompaniments this is a nutritionally complete meal—three servings of vegetables, your full day's supply of vitamin C, plenty of minerals, and polyphenols from the pomegranates and walnuts.

Per serving: 37g protein, 87g carbohydrate, 28g fat, 19g fiber, 708 calories/2973 kJ

Chile con Carne with Peanuts

You may think this won't be enough meat for four, but with the addition of peanuts it makes a satisfying dinner. The whole peanuts add an unusual crunchy texture to this old favorite.

SERVES 4

½ tablespoon extra-virgin
  olive oil

1 onion, chopped

2 small (hot) fresh red chiles,
  seeded and chopped

3 cloves garlic, chopped

1 teaspoon cumin seeds, coarsely
  pounded in a mortar and pestle

9 ounces lean ground beef

1¾ cups shelled peanuts

1 cup canned or cooked
  red kidney beans

One 14-ounce can chopped
  tomatoes

2¼ cups chicken stock

Salt and freshly ground
  black pepper

PREHEAT the oven to 275°F.

WARM the oil in a large skillet over low heat. Add the onion and cook until slightly softened. Add the chiles and garlic and cook for 2 to 3 minutes, until softened. Add the cumin and cook an additional minute or two, until fragrant. Remove the onion, chiles, and garlic with a slotted spoon and put them in an ovenproof casserole. Raise the heat and brown the beef in the skillet, then add it to the casserole.

PROCESS half the peanuts to fine crumbs in a food processor and add to the casserole; add the whole peanuts, too, along with the kidney beans, tomatoes (with their juice), and stock. Mix well, cover, place in the oven, and cook for about 2½ hours, until the sauce thickens, checking and stirring once or twice. Season with salt and pepper to taste. Serve with brown rice and a large green salad.

It's a good idea to include more plant protein in your diet: Less meat and more nuts! This also reduces the saturated fat content of your food. This dish is a good source of useful minerals, with about half your daily iron, magnesium, and zinc requirements.

Per serving: 39g protein, 54g carbohydrate, 37g fat, 13g fiber, 675 calories/2835 kJ

Pork Tenderloin with Spicy Mashed Persimmons

When buying pork, always choose the best-quality free-range meat—it has a superior flavor, is better for the pigs, and better for you.

SERVES 4

FOR THE SPICY MASHED
PERSIMMONS:

*1-inch piece fresh ginger, peeled
    and roughly chopped*
2 cloves garlic, peeled
*1 large red onion, roughly
    chopped*
*1 red bell pepper, seeded
    and roughly chopped*
1 small hot red chile, seeded
½ teaspoon cumin seeds

4 or 5 cardamom pods
1 tablespoon extra-virgin olive oil
4 ounces ripe tomatoes
*3 persimmons, leaves and bases
    removed (but do not peel),
    roughly chopped*
Juice of 1 lime
*Salt and freshly ground
    black pepper*
1 pound pork tenderloin
1 teaspoon extra-virgin olive oil

IN a food processor, process the ginger, garlic, onion, bell pepper, and chile with 1 tablespoon water. Pound the cumin seeds and black seeds from the cardamom pods lightly with a mortar and pestle. Put the oil in a casserole and warm over low heat. Sauté the pounded spices for a minute or two, then add the blended mixture and cook, stirring, for about 10 minutes. Place the tomatoes and persimmons in a food processor and process well. Add this mixture and the lime juice to the casserole, stir, turn the heat down, cover, and cook for 30 minutes to 1 hour, until smooth and soft, stirring and adding a little more water when necessary to prevent sticking. Season with salt and pepper to taste.

WHILE the persimmons are cooking, cut the pork into 4 portions and brush lightly with olive oil. Grill on both sides until the meat is cooked through (about 10 minutes on each side, depending on the thickness of the meat and the heat of your grill). Serve the pork on a bed of the mashed persimmons, with a green vegetable such as steamed spinach.

NUTRITIONAL BENEFITS

Tenderloin is a lean cut of pork, which keeps the saturated fat content down. Pork is a good source of B-group vitamins, especially thiamin.

Per serving: 28g protein, 15g carbohydrate, 9g fat, 2g fiber, 249 calories/1045 kJ

Beef Stew with Cranberries

Like most stews, this is best prepared a day ahead; the meat will be more tender and you can lift off the solid fat for a much cleaner tasting and healthier dish.

serves 4

1 tablespoon extra-virgin olive oil

1½ pounds lean braising beef

1¼ pounds baby onions

10 ounces carrots, chopped

3 celery stalks, sliced

2 red bell peppers, sliced

3 cloves garlic, crushed

4 bay leaves

2 cups beef or vegetable stock

Salt and freshly ground black pepper

2 cups fresh or frozen cranberries

PREHEAT the oven to 325°F.

HEAT the oil in a heat-proof casserole over medium-high heat, add the meat, and brown quickly on all sides. Remove to a plate. Add the onions, carrots, celery, red bell peppers, and garlic and cook, stirring frequently, for about 5 minutes, or until softened. Return the meat to the casserole, along with the bay leaves and stock, bring to a simmer, then place in the oven for about 1½ hours, until the meat is tender. Remove from the oven, cool, then refrigerate overnight.

THE next day, remove the fat that has solidified on top of the casserole and the bay leaves. Reheat in the oven or on top of the stove. Season with salt and pepper to taste. Add the cranberries and simmer for an additional 15 to 20 minutes.

SERVE with broccoli and new potatoes boiled in their skins.

LAMB TAGINE WITH CRANBERRIES

USE lean lamb instead of the beef; add 1 teaspoon ground cinnamon, 1 teaspoon ground cumin, 1 teaspoon paprika, and 2 teaspoons grated fresh ginger to the vegetables. Serve with Walnut Pilaf (page 250).

NUTRITIONAL BENEFITS

Cranberries add both procyanidins and vitamin C to the stew. This dish is also a rich source of beta-carotene, lutein, and zeaxanthin, plus a full range of vitamins and minerals—including two thirds of your daily zinc.

Per serving (with 4 ounces broccoli and 4 ounces new potatoes: 41g protein, 62g carbohydrate, 10g fat, 13g fiber, 489 calories/2052 kJ

STIR-FRIED LIVER

A colorful supper that's quick and easy to make

SERVES 4

3½ ounces black beans,
    soaked overnight

1 tablespoon extra-virgin olive oil

1 large onion or 6 scallions,
    chopped

2 cloves garlic, chopped

1-inch piece of fresh ginger,
    chopped

1 red bell pepper, sliced

1 green bell pepper, sliced

4 ounces mushrooms, sliced

4 ounces bean sprouts, rinsed

9 ounces lamb's liver, cut into strips

⅓ cup red wine

2 tablespoons soy sauce
    (preferably tamari)

2 tablespoons tomato purée

Freshly ground black pepper

DRAIN the soaked beans, place in a saucepan, cover with cold water—do not add salt—and bring to a boil for 10 minutes. Reduce the heat and simmer for 30 to 50 minutes, until tender. Drain well.

HEAT the oil in a wok or large nonstick skillet over medium-high heat. Add the onion, garlic, and ginger and stir-fry until the onion is translucent, about 3 minutes. Add the bell peppers and mushrooms and stir-fry until the peppers begin to soften; about 3 to 5 minutes.

ADD the beans, bean sprouts, and liver, stirring well with each addition so that it doesn't stick. Add the wine, stir briefly, then add the soy sauce, tomato purée, and pepper to taste and stir-fry for an additional 2 to 3 minutes to warm through.

SERVE with brown rice.

NUTRITIONAL BENEFITS

With enough vitamin B_{12} to last for 3 weeks, this is also an excellent source of vitamin C and other B vitamins, magnesium, zinc, and iron.

Per serving (with ½ cup rice): 24g protein, 51g carbohydrate, 8g fat, 8g fiber, 382 calories/ 1604 kJ

Chocolate Truffle "Ice Cream"

My frozen chocolate dessert is made with no added sugar—it has an intensely chocolaty taste. Lecithin—available from health food stores—is an emulsifier that gives nondairy frozen desserts a smooth texture.

serves 16

2 small ripe pears, peeled
   and cored

⅔ cup dried dates

2 tablespoons water

1 medium banana, cut into pieces

3.5 ounces unsweetened
   cocoa powder

1 cup orange juice (juice of
   3 large oranges)

2 tablespoons canola oil
   or walnut oil

2 teaspoons vanilla extract

2 teaspoons lecithin
   (optional)

PLACE the pears, dates, and water in a nonstick saucepan over low heat. Cover and cook 15 to 20 minutes, until soft. Remove the lid and leave to cool, then purée in a blender. Add the banana and blend until smooth.

WHILE the pears are cooking, mix the cocoa and orange juice to make a smooth paste, then stir in the oil, vanilla, and lecithin, if using. Add the cocoa mixture to the pear and date mixture, and blend until smooth. Transfer to a sealable freezerproof container and freeze for at least 4 hours.

To serve, remove from the freezer and leave to soften at room temperature for 30 minutes. Serve with strawberries or raspberries.

NUTRITIONAL BENEFITS

This rich-tasting vegan dessert contains procyanidins from the cocoa and vitamin C from the orange juice, and has a low glycemic load.

Per serving: 2g protein, 14g carbohydrate, 3g fat, 3g fiber, 68 calories/285 kJ

CRANBERRY AND APPLE CRUMBLE

Use as much cinnamon as you like—it brings out the sweetness of the apples.

SERVES 6

1 cup fresh or frozen cranberries
14 ounces apples, peeled, cored,
*   and roughly chopped*
Grated zest and juice of 1 orange
½ cup rolled oats
Scant ½ cup whole-wheat flour

5 tablespoons unsalted butter,
*   chilled, chopped into small pieces*
⅓ cup turbinado sugar
1 to 2 teaspoons ground
*   cinnamon*
⅔ cup finely chopped walnuts

PREHEAT the oven to 400°F.

COMBINE the cranberries, apples, and orange zest and juice in a baking dish.

IN a large bowl, lightly rub together the oats, flour, and butter until they form even crumbs. Stir in the sugar, cinnamon, and walnuts. Spoon the mixture over the fruits, spreading it evenly right to the edge of the dish.

Bake for 30 to 35 minutes, until the top is nicely browned. Serve hot, with a dollop of thick Greek yogurt.

NUTRITIONAL BENEFITS

Apples, cranberries, and cinnamon are all good sources of procyanidins; walnuts contain other beneficial polyphenols.

Per serving: *5g protein, 37g carbohydrate, 18g fat, 5g fiber, 312 calories/1310 kJ*

appendix
FIND YOUR BODY mass index (BMI)

Doctors, nutritionists, and other health professionals use the Body Mass Index (BMI) to gauge an adult's weight-related health risk. The BMI is a ratio of height to weight, and it's a fairly accurate standard for determining whether someone is at a healthy weight or is overweight and at risk of weight-related problems such as high blood pressure and diabetes.

Take a look at either the imperial or metric version of the chart to calculate your BMI. Find your height in the left-hand column, then move across that row to find the number closest to your weight. Now follow that column to the bottom of the chart, where you'll find your BMI.

If you want to calculate your BMI more accurately, for the imperial system, multiply your weight in pounds by 703, then divide by your height in inches squared. For the metric system, divide your weight (in kilograms) by your height (in meters) squared. Here's where you stand:

BMI below 18.5   underweight
BMI 18.5–24.9   normal
BMI 25–30   overweight
BMI over 30   obese

A BMI between 18.5 and 24.9 is generally considered healthy, although you should also take into account other risk factors, including your age, level of physical activity, eating habits, and family history.

YOUR BODY MASS INDEX (BMI)—IMPERIAL

HEIGHT (FEET, INCHES)	WEIGHT (POUNDS)													
4'10"	91	96	100	105	110	115	119	124	129	134	139	143	148	153
4'11"	94	99	104	109	114	119	124	128	133	138	143	148	153	158
5'0"	97	102	107	112	118	123	128	133	138	143	148	153	158	163
5'1"	100	106	111	116	122	127	132	137	143	148	153	158	164	169
5'2"	104	109	115	120	126	131	136	142	147	153	158	164	169	174
5'3"	107	113	118	124	130	135	141	146	152	158	163	169	175	180
5'4"	110	116	122	128	134	140	145	151	157	163	169	174	180	186
5'5"	114	120	126	132	138	144	150	156	162	168	174	180	186	192
5'6"	118	124	130	136	142	148	155	161	167	173	179	186	192	198
5'7"	121	127	134	140	146	153	159	166	172	178	185	191	197	204
5'8"	125	131	138	144	151	158	164	171	177	184	190	197	203	210
5'9"	128	135	142	149	155	162	169	176	182	189	196	203	209	216
5'10"	132	139	146	153	160	167	174	181	188	195	202	207	215	222
5'11"	136	142	150	157	165	172	179	186	193	200	208	213	222	229
6'0"	140	147	154	162	169	177	184	191	199	206	213	221	228	235
6'1"	144	151	158	166	175	182	190	197	204	212	219	227	234	242
6'2"	148	155	163	171	179	186	194	202	210	218	226	233	241	249
6'3"	152	160	168	176	184	192	200	208	216	224	232	240	248	256
6'4"	156	163	172	180	188	197	205	213	221	230	238	246	254	262
6'5"	160	168	177	185	194	202	210	219	227	236	244	252	261	269
6'6"	164	173	181	190	199	207	216	225	233	242	250	259	268	276
BMI	19	20	21	22	23	24	25	26	27	28	29	30	31	32

YOUR BODY MASS INDEX (BMI)—METRIC

WEIGHT (KILOGRAMS)

HEIGHT (METERS)														
1.48	42	44	46	48	50	53	55	57	59	61	64	66	68	70
1.50	43	45	47	50	52	54	56	59	61	63	65	68	70	72
1.52	44	46	49	51	53	55	58	60	62	65	67	69	72	74
1.54	45	47	50	52	55	57	59	62	64	66	69	71	74	76
1.56	46	49	51	54	56	58	61	63	66	68	71	73	75	78
1.58	47	50	52	55	57	60	62	65	67	70	72	75	77	80
1.60	49	51	54	56	59	61	64	67	69	72	74	77	79	82
1.62	50	53	55	58	60	63	66	68	71	74	77	80	82	85
1.64	51	54	57	60	62	65	67	70	73	75	78	81	83	86
1.66	52	55	58	61	63	66	69	72	74	77	80	83	85	88
1.68	54	56	59	62	65	68	71	73	76	79	82	85	88	90
1.70	55	58	61	64	67	69	72	75	78	81	84	87	90	93
1.72	56	59	62	65	68	71	74	77	80	83	86	89	92	95
1.74	58	61	64	67	70	73	76	79	82	85	88	91	94	97
1.76	59	62	65	68	71	73	77	80	84	87	90	93	96	99
1.78	60	63	67	70	73	76	79	82	86	89	92	95	98	101
1.80	62	65	68	71	75	78	81	84	88	91	94	97	100	104
1.82	63	66	70	73	76	80	83	86	89	93	96	100	103	106
1.84	64	68	71	75	78	81	85	88	91	95	98	102	105	108
1.86	66	69	73	76	80	83	87	90	93	97	100	104	107	111
1.88	67	70	74	78	81	84	88	92	95	99	102	106	109	113
1.90	69	72	76	79	83	87	90	94	98	101	105	108	111	116
1.92	70	74	77	81	85	89	92	96	100	103	107	111	114	118
1.94	72	75	79	83	87	90	94	98	102	105	109	113	117	120
1.96	73	77	81	85	88	92	96	100	104	108	111	115	119	123
1.98	75	78	82	87	90	94	98	102	106	110	114	118	122	126
2.00	76	80	84	88	92	96	100	104	108	112	116	120	124	128
BMI	19	20	21	22	23	24	25	26	27	28	29	30	31	32

references

CHAPTER 2: WINE AND HEALTH

Anderson, J. C., Alpern, Z., Sethi, G., et al., "Prevalence and risk of colorectal neoplasia in consumers of alcohol in a screening population," *Am J Gastroenterol* 2005; 100: 2049–55.

Barstad, B., Sorensen, T. I., Tjonneland, A., et al., "Intake of wine, beer and spirits and risk of gastric cancer," *Eur J Cancer Prev* 2005; 14: 239–43.

Britton, A., Singh-Manoux, A., Marmot, M., "Alcohol consumption and cognitive function in the Whitehall II Study," *Am J Epidemiol* 2004; 160: 240–7.

Choi, H. K., Atkinson, K., Karlson, E. W., Willett, W., Curhan, G., "Alcohol intake and risk of incident gout in men: a prospective study," *Lancet* 2004; 363: 1277–81.

Choi, H. K., "Dietary risk factors for rheumatic diseases," *Curr Opin Rheumatol* 2005; 17: 141–6.

Colditz, G. A., Rosner, B., "Cumulative risk of breast cancer to age 70 years according to risk factor status: data from the Nurses' Health Study," *Am J Epidemiol* 2000; 152: 950–64.

de Lorgeril, M., Renaud, S., Mamelle, N., et al., "Mediterranean alpha-linolenic acid-rich diet in secondary prevention of coronary heart disease," *Lancet* 1994; 343: 1454–9.

de Lorgeril, M., Salen, P., Martin, J. L., et al., "Wine drinking and risks of cardiovascular complications after recent acute myocardial infarction," *Circulation* 2002; 106: 1465–9.

de Lorgeril, M., Salen, P., Martin, J. L., et al., "Mediterranean diet, traditional risk factors, and the rate of cardiovascular complications after myocardial infarction: final report of the Lyon Diet Heart Study," *Circulation* 1999; 99: 779–85.

Djousse, L., Arnett, D. K., Eckfeldt, J. H., et al., "Alcohol consumption and metabolic syndrome: does the type of beverage matter?" *Obes Res* 2004; 12: 1375–85.

Djousse, L., Levy, D., Murabito, J. M., Cupples, L. A., Ellison, R. C., "Alcohol consumption and risk of intermittent claudication in the Framingham Heart Study," *Circulation* 2000; 102: 3092–7.

Ellison, R. C., Zhang, Y., McLennan, C. E., Rothman, K. J., "Exploring the relation of alcohol consumption to risk of breast cancer," *Am J Epidemiol* 2001; 154: 740–7.

Gronbaek, M., Becker, U., Johansen, D., et al., "Type of alcohol consumed and mortality from all causes, coronary heart disease, and cancer," *Ann Intern Med* 2000; 133: 411–9.

Hendriks, H. F., Veenstra, J., Velthuis-te Wierik, E. J., Schaafsma, G., Kluft, C., "Effect of moderate dose of alcohol with evening meal on fibrinolytic factors," *BMJ* 1994; 308: 1003–6.

Howard, A. A., Arnsten, J. H., Gourevitch, M. N., "Effect of alcohol consumption on diabetes mellitus: a systematic review," *Ann Intern Med* 2004; 140: 211–9.

Klatsky, A. L., Friedman, G. D., Armstrong, M. A., Kipp, H., "Wine, liquor, beer, and mortality," *Am J Epidemiol* 2003; 158: 585–95.

Larrieu, S., Letenneur, L., Helmer, C., Dartigues, J. F., Barberger-Gateau, P., "Nutritional factors and risk of incident dementia in the PAQUID longitudinal cohort," *J Nutr Health Aging* 2004; 8: 150–4.

Lukasiewicz, E., Mennen, L. I., Bertrais, S., et al., "Alcohol intake in relation to body mass index and waist-to-hip ratio: the importance of type of alcoholic beverage," *Public Health Nutr* 2005; 8: 315–20.

Mukamal, K. J., Ascherio, A., Mittleman, M. A., et al., "Alcohol and risk for ischemic stroke in men: the role of drinking patterns and usual beverage," *Ann Intern Med* 2005; 142: 11–9.

Mukamal, K. J., Conigrave, K. M., Mittleman, M. A., et al., "Roles of drinking pattern and type of alcohol consumed in coronary heart disease in men," *N Engl J Med* 2003; 348: 109–18.

Mukamal, K. J., Kuller, L. H., Fitzpatrick, A. L., et al., "Prospective study of alcohol consumption and risk of dementia in older adults," *JAMA* 2003; 289: 1405–13.

Norrie, P., *Wine & Health. A new look at an old medicine*. Apollo Books (published by C. Pierson, Mosman, NSW 2088, Australia).

Obisesan, T. O., Hirsch, R., Kosoko, O., Carlson, L., Parrott, M., "Moderate wine consumption is associated with decreased odds of developing age-related macular degeneration in NHANES-1," *J Am Geriatr Soc* 1998; 46: 1–7.

Platz, E. A., Leitzmann, M. F., Rimm, E. B., Willett, W. C., Giovannucci, E., "Alcohol intake, drinking patterns, and risk of prostate cancer in a large prospective cohort study," *Am J Epidemiol* 2004; 159: 444–53.

Renaud, S., de Lorgeril, M. "Wine, alcohol, platelets, and the French paradox for coronary heart disease," *Lancet* 1992; 339: 1523–6.

Renaud, S. C., Gueguen, R., Siest, G., Salamon, R., "Wine, beer, and mortality in middle-aged men from eastern France," *Arch Intern Med* 1999; 159: 1865–70.

Rimm, E. B., Klatsky, A., Grobbee, D., Stampfer, M. J., "Review of moderate alcohol consumption and reduced risk of coronary heart disease: is the effect due to beer, wine, or spirits?" *BMJ* 1996; 312: 731–6.

Ruidavets, J. B., Bataille, V., Dallongeville, J., et al., "Alcohol intake and diet in France, the prominent role of lifestyle," *Eur Heart J* 2004; 25: 1153–62.

St. Leger, A. S., Cochrane, A. L., Moore, F., "Factors associated with cardiac mortality in developed countries with particular reference to the consumption of wine," *Lancet* 1979; 1: 1017–20.

Schroder, H., Marrugat, J., Vila, J., Covas, M. I., Elosua, R., "Adherence to the traditional Mediterranean diet is inversely associated with body mass index and obesity in a Spanish population," *J Nutr* 2004; 134: 3355–61.

Siler, S. Q., Neese, R. A., Christiansen, M. P., Hellerstein, M. K., "The inhibition of gluconeogenesis following alcohol in humans," *Am J Physiol* 1998; 275: E897–907.

Stampfer, M. J., Kang, J. H., Chen, J., Cherry, R., Grodstein, F., "Effects of moderate alcohol consumption on cognitive function in women," *N Engl J Med* 2005; 352: 245–53.

Tjonneland, A., Gronbaek, M., Stripp, C., Overvad, K., "Wine intake and diet in a random sample of 48,763 Danish men and women," *Am J Clin Nutr* 1999; 69: 49–54.

Truelsen, T., Thudium, D., Gronbaek, M., "Copenhagen City Heart Study. Amount and type of alcohol and risk of dementia: the Copenhagen City Heart Study," *Neurology* 2002; 59: 1313–9.

Vliegenthart, R., Geleijnse, J. M., Hofman, A., et al., "Alcohol consumption and risk of peripheral arterial disease: the Rotterdam study," *Am J Epidemiol* 2002; 155: 332–8.

Yusuf, S., Hawken, S., Ounpuu, S., et al., "Effect of potentially modifiable risk factors associated with myocardial infarction in 52 countries (the INTERHEART study): case-control study," *Lancet* 2004; 364: 937-52.

CHAPTER 3: WHAT IS IT ABOUT RED WINE?

Auger, C., Teissedre, P. L., Gerain, P., et al., "Dietary wine phenolics catechin, quercetin, and resveratrol efficiently protect hypercholesterolemic hamsters against aortic fatty streak accumulation," *J Agric Food Chem* 2005; 53: 2015–21.

Blanco-Colio, L. M., Valderrama, M., Alvarez-Sala, L. A., et al., "Red wine intake prevents nuclear factor-kappaB activation in peripheral blood mononuclear cells of healthy volunteers during postprandial lipemia," *Circulation* 2000; 102: 1020–6.

Corder, R., Douthwaite, J. A., Lees, D. M., et al., "Endothelin-1 synthesis reduced by red wine," *Nature* 2001; 414: 863–4.

de Rijke, Y. B., Demacker, P. N., Assen, N. A., et al., "Red wine consumption does not affect oxidizability of low-density lipoproteins in volunteers," *Am J Clin Nutr* 1996; 63: 329–34.

Estruch, R., Sacanella, E., Badia, E., et al., "Different effects of red wine and gin consumption on inflammatory biomarkers of atherosclerosis: a prospective randomized crossover trial. Effects of wine on inflammatory markers," *Atherosclerosis* 2004; 175: 117–23.

Fitzpatrick, D. F., Bing, B., Maggi, D. A., Fleming, R. C., O'Malley, R. M., "Vasodilating procyanidins derived from grape seeds," *NY Acad Sci* 2002; 957: 78–89.

Fitzpatrick, D. F., Hirschfield, S. L., Coffey, R. G., "Endothelium-dependent vasorelaxing activity of wine and other grape products," *Am J Physiol* 1993; 265: H774–8.

Frankel, E. N., Kanner, J., German, J. B., Parks, E., Kinsella, J. E. "Inhibition of oxidation of human low-density lipoprotein by phenolic substances in red wine," *Lancet* 1993; 341: 454–7.

Frankel, E. N., Waterhouse, A. L., Kinsella, J. E., "Inhibition of human LDL oxidation by resveratrol," *Lancet* 1993; 341: 1103–4.

Freedman, J. E., Parker, C. 3rd, Li, L., et al., "Select flavonoids and whole juice from purple grapes inhibit platelet function and enhance nitric oxide release," *Circulation* 2001; 103: 2792–8.

Gehm, B. D., McAndrews, J. M., Chien, P. Y., Jameson, J. L., "Resveratrol, a polyphenolic compound found in grapes and wine, is an agonist for the estrogen receptor," *Proc Natl Acad Sci USA* 1997; 94: 14138–43.

Goldberg, D. M., Yan, J., Soleas, G. J., "Absorption of three wine-related polyphenols in three different matrices by healthy subjects," *Clin Biochem* 2003; 36: 79–87.

Gryglewski, R. J., Korbut, R., Robak, J., Swies, J., "On the mechanism of antithrombotic action of flavonoids," *Biochem Pharmacol.* 1987; 36: 317–22.

Hashimoto, M., Kim, S., Eto, M., et al., "Effect of acute intake of red wine on flow-mediated vasodilatation of the brachial artery," *Am J Cardiol* 2001; 88: 1457–60.

Jang, M., Cai, L., Udeani, G. O., et al., "Cancer chemopreventive activity of resveratrol, a natural product derived from grapes," *Science* 1997; 275: 218–20.

Kopp, P., "Resveratrol, a phytoestrogen found in red wine, A possible explanation for the conundrum of the 'French paradox'?" *Eur J Endocrinol* 1998; 138: 619–20.

Klurfeld, D. M., Kritchevsky, D., "Differential effects of alcoholic beverages on experimental atherosclerosis in rabbits," *Exp Mol Pathol* 1981; 34: 62–71.

Nigdikar, S. V., Williams, N. R., Griffin, B. A., Howard, A. N., "Consumption of red wine polyphenols reduces the susceptibility of low-density lipoproteins to oxidation in vivo," *Am J Clin Nutr* 1998; 68: 258-65.

Pace-Asciak, C. R., Hahn, S., Diamandis, E. P., Soleas, G., Goldberg, D. M., "The red wine phenolics trans-resveratrol and quercetin block human platelet aggregation and eicosanoid synthesis: implications for protection against coronary heart disease," *Clin Chim Acta* 1995; 235: 207–19.

Siemann, E. H., Creasy, L. L., "Concentration of the phytoalexin resveratrol in wine," *Am J Enol Vitic* 1992; 43: 49–52.

Soleas, G. J., Diamandis, E. P., Goldberg, D. M., "Resveratrol: a molecule whose time has come? And gone?" *Clin Biochem* 1997; 30: 91–113.

Stein, J. H., Keevil, J. G., Wiebe, D. A., Aeschlimann, S., Folts, J. D., "Purple grape juice improves endothelial function and reduces the susceptibility of LDL cholesterol to oxidation in patients with coronary artery disease," *Circulation* 1999; 100: 1050–5.

Vinson, J. A., Teufel, K., Wu, N., "Red wine, dealcoholized red wine, and especially grape juice, inhibit atherosclerosis in a hamster model," *Atherosclerosis* 2001; 156: 67–72.

Yamakoshi, J., Kataoka, S., Koga, T., Ariga, T., "Proanthocyanidin-rich extract from grape seeds attenuates the development of aortic atherosclerosis in cholesterol-fed rabbits," *Atherosclerosis* 1999; 142: 139–49.

Chapter 4: The Magic of Procyanidins

Aviram, M., Dornfeld, L., Rosenblat, M., et al., "Pomegranate juice consumption reduces oxidative stress, atherogenic modifications to LDL, and platelet aggregation: studies in humans and in atherosclerotic apolipoprotein E-deficient mice," *Am J Clin Nutr* 2000; 71: 1062–76.

Buijsse, B., Feskens, E. J., Kok, F. J., Kromhout, D., "Cocoa intake, blood pressure, and cardiovascular mortality: the Zutphen Elderly Study," *Arch Intern Med* 2006; 166: 411–7.

Chevaux, K. A., Schmitz, H. H., Romanczyk, L. J. Jr., "Food products containing polyphenol(s) and L-arginine to stimulate nitric oxide," U.S. Patent 6,805,883.

Duffy, S. J., Keaney, J. F. Jr, Holbrook, M., et al., "Short- and long-term black tea consumption reverses endothelial dysfunction in patients with coronary artery disease," *Circulation* 2001; 104: 151–6.

Fisher, N. D., Hughes, M., Gerhard-Herman, M., Hollenberg, N. K., "Flavanol-rich cocoa induces nitric-oxide-dependent vasodilation in healthy humans," *J Hypertens* 2003; 21: 2281–6.

Fukuda, T., Ito, H., Yoshida, T., "Antioxidative polyphenols from walnuts (Juglans regia L.)," *Phytochemistry* 2003; 63: 795–801.

Grassi, D., Necozione, S., Lippi, C., et al., "Cocoa reduces blood pressure and insulin resistance and improves endothelium-dependent vasodilation in hypertensives," *Hypertension* 2005; 46: 398–405.

Hammerstone, J. F., Lazarus, S. A., Mitchell, A. E., Rucker, R., Schmitz, H. H., "Identification of procyanidins in cocoa (Theobroma cacao) and chocolate using high-performance liquid chromatography/mass spectrometry," *J Agric Food Chem* 1999; 47: 490–6.

Hammerstone, J. F., Lazarus, S. A., Schmitz, H. H., "Procyanidin content and variation in some commonly consumed foods," *J Nutr* 2000; 130 (8S Suppl): 2086S–92S.

Hollenberg, N. K., Martinez, G., McCullough, M., et al., "Aging, acculturation, salt intake, and hypertension in the Kuna of Panama," *Hypertension* 1997; 29: 171–6

Karim, M., McCormick, K., Kappagoda, C. T., "Effects of cocoa extracts on endothelium-dependent relaxation," *J Nutr* 2000; 130 (8S Suppl): 2105S–8S.

Kealey, K. S., Snyder, R. M., Romanczyk, L. J. Jr., et al., "Procyanidin-L-arginine combinations," U.S. Patent Application 20030215558.

Lee, K. W., Kim, Y. J., Lee, H. J., Lee, C. Y. "Cocoa has more phenolic phytochemicals and a higher antioxidant capacity than teas and red wine," *J Agric Food Chem* 2003; 51: 7292–5.

Malik, A., Afaq, F., Sarfaraz, S., et al., "Pomegranate fruit juice for chemoprevention and chemotherapy of prostate cancer," *Proc Natl Acad Sci USA* 2005; 102: 14813–8.

Mullen, W., McGinn, J., Lean, M. E., et al., "Ellagitannins, flavonoids, and other phenolics in red raspberries and their contribution to antioxidant capacity and vasorelaxation properties," *J Agric Food Chem* 2002; 50: 5191–6.

Peters, U., Poole, C., Arab, L., "Does tea affect cardiovascular disease? A meta-analysis," *Am J Epidemiol* 2001; 154: 495–503.

Ramljak, D., Romanczyk, L. J., Metheny-Barlow, L. J., et al., "Pentameric procyanidin from Theobroma cacao selectively inhibits growth of human breast cancer cells," *Mol Cancer Ther* 2005; 4: 537–46.

Ros, E., Nunez, I., Perez-Heras, A., et al., "A walnut diet improves endothelial function in hypercholesterolemic subjects: a randomized crossover trial," *Circulation* 2004; 109: 1609–14.

Sabate, J., "Nut consumption, vegetarian diets, ischemic heart disease risk, and all-cause mortality: evidence from epidemiologic studies," *Am J Clin Nutr* 1999; 70 (3 Suppl): 500S–503S.

Schroeter, H., Heiss, C., Balzer, J., et al., "(-)-Epicatechin mediates beneficial effects of flavanol-rich cocoa on vascular function in humans," *Proc Natl Acad Sci USA* 2006; 103: 1024–9.

Sumner, M. D., Elliott-Eller, M., Weidner, G., et al., "Effects of pomegranate juice consumption on myocardial perfusion in patients with coronary heart disease," *Am J Cardiol* 2005; 96: 810–4.

Uchida, S., Ohta, H., Niwa, M., et al., "Prolongation of life span of stroke-prone spontaneously hypertensive rats (SHRSP) ingesting persimmon tannin," *Chem Pharm Bull* (Tokyo) 1990; 38: 1049–52.

USDA Database for the Proanthocyanidin Content of Selected Foods—2004.

Vita, J. A., "Tea consumption and cardiovascular disease: effects on endothelial function," *J Nutr* 2003; 133: 3293S–7S.

Vlachopoulos, C., Aznaouridis, K., Alexopoulos, N., et al., "Effect of dark chocolate on arterial function in healthy individuals," *Am J Hypertens* 2005; 18: 785–91.

Vrhovsek, U., Rigo, A., Tonon, D., Mattivi, F., "Quantitation of polyphenols in different apple varieties," *J Agric Food Chem* 2004; 52: 6532–8.

CHAPTER 5: DO SIMILAR NATURAL REMEDIES WORK?

David, R., Masquelier, J., "La localisation des composés catéchiques phlorogluciques dans les organes végétatifs du Pin maritime," *C. R. Hebd Seances Acad Sci* 1952; 235: 1325–7.

Gabor, M., "Szent-Gyorgyi and the bioflavonoids: new results and perspectives of pharmacological research into benzo-pyrone derivatives," Commemoration on the 50th anniversary of the award of the Nobel Prize, *Prog Clin Biol Res* 1988; 280: 1–15.

Lalukota, K., Cleland, J. G., Ingle, L., Clark, A. L., Coletta, A. P., "Clinical trials update from the Heart Failure Society of America: EMOTE, HERB-CHF, BEST genetic sub-study and RHYTHM-ICD," *Eur J Heart Fail* 2004; 6: 953–5.

Masquelier, J., "Plant extract with a proanthocyanidins content as therapeutic agent having radical scavenger effect and use thereof," U.S. Patent No. 4,698,360.

Masquelier, J., "Identification et dosage des facteurs vitaminiques P dans diverses boissons fermentées," *Bull Soc Chim Biol* (Paris) 1956; 38: 65–70.

Masquelier, J., "Le vin dans l'alimentation," *Aliment Vie* 1965; 53: 261–70.

Masquelier, J., Michaud, J., Laparra, J., Dumon, M. C., "Flavonoides et pycnogenols," *Int J Vitam Nutr Res* 1979; 49: 307–11.

Rohdewald, P. "Method of controlling the reactivity of human blood platelets by oral administration of the extract of the maritime pine (pycnogenol)," U.S. Patent No. 5,720,956.

Tauchert, M., "Efficacy and safety of crataegus extract WS 1442 in comparison with placebo in patients with chronic stable New York Heart Association class-III heart failure," *Am Heart J* 2002; 143: 910–5.

Chapter 6: Eat, Drink, and Be Healthy at 100 Years Old

Baibas, N., Trichopoulou, A., Voridis, E., Trichopoulos, D., "Residence in mountainous compared with lowland areas in relation to total and coronary mortality. A study in rural Greece," *J Epidemiol Community Health* 2005; 59: 274–8.

Berrigan, D., Perkins, S. N., Haines, D. C., Hursting, S. D., "Adult-onset calorie restriction and fasting delay spontaneous tumorigenesis in p53-deficient mice," *Carcinogenesis* 2002; 23: 817–22.

Coles, L. S., "Demography of human supercentenarians," *J Gerontol A Biol Sci Med Sci* 2004; 59: B579–86.

Deiana, L., Ferrucci, L., Pes, G. M., et al., "AKEntAnnos. The Sardinia Study of Extreme Longevity," *Aging* (Milano) 1999; 11: 142–9.

Dirks, A. J., Leeuwenburgh, C., "Caloric restriction in humans: potential pitfalls and health concerns," *Mech Ageing Dev* 2006; 127: 1–7.

Evert, J., Lawler, E., Bogan, H., Perls, T., "Morbidity profiles of centenarians: survivors, delayers, and escapers," *J Gerontol A Biol Sci Med Sci* 2003; 58: 232–7.

Farchi, G., Fidanza, F., Giampaoli, S., Mariotti, S., Menotti, A., "Alcohol and survival in the Italian rural cohorts of the Seven Countries Study," *Int J Epidemiol* 2000; 29: 667–71.

Fontana, L., Meyer, T. E., Klein, S., Holloszy, J. O., "Long-term calorie restriction is highly effective in reducing the risk for atherosclerosis in humans," *Proc Natl Acad Sci USA* 2004; 101: 6659–63.

Keys, A., Aravanis, C., Blackburn, H., et al., "Probability of Middle-Aged Men Developing Coronary Heart Disease in Five Years," *Circulation* 1972; 45: 815–28.

Keys, A., Menotti, A., Karvonen, M. J., et al., "The diet and 15-year death rate in the Seven Countries Study," *Am J Epidemiol* 1986; 124: 903–15.

Kromhout, D., Keys, A., Aravanis, C., et al., "Food consumption patterns in the 1960s in seven countries," *Am J Clin Nutr* 1989; 49: 889–94.

Lee, I. M., Manson, J. E., Hennekens, C. H., Paffenbarger, R. S. Jr., "Body weight and mortality. A 27-year follow-up of middle-aged men," *JAMA* 1993; 270: 2823–8.

Manson, J. E., Willett, W. C., Stampfer, M. J., et al., "Body weight and mortality among women," *N Engl J Med* 1995; 333: 677–85.

Menotti, A., Keys, A., Kromhout, D., et al., "Inter-cohort differences in coronary heart disease mortality in the 25-year follow-up of the Seven Countries Study," *Eur J Epidemiol* 1993; 9: 527–36.

Mimura, G., Murakami, K., Gushiken, M., "Nutritional factors for longevity in Okinawa—present and future," *Nutr Health* 1992; 8: 159–63.

Moschandreas, J., Kafatos, A., Aravanis, C., et al., "Long-term predictors of survival for the Seven Countries Study cohort from Crete: from 1960 to 2000," *Int J Cardiol* 2005; 100: 85–91.

Nasir, K., Raggi, P., Rumberger, J. A., et al., "Coronary artery calcium volume scores on electron beam tomography in 12,936 asymptomatic adults," *Am J Cardiol* 2004; 93: 1146–9.

Perls, T. T., Wilmoth, J., Levenson, R., et al., "Life-long sustained mortality advantage of siblings of centenarians," *Proc Natl Acad Sci USA* 2002; 99: 8442–7.

Poulain, M., Pes, G. M., Grasland, C., et al., "Identification of a geographic area characterized by extreme longevity in the Sardinia island: the AKEA study," *Exp Gerontol* 2004; 39: 1423–9.

Rumberger, J. A., Kaufman, L., "A rosetta stone for coronary calcium risk stratification: Agatston, volume, and mass scores in 11,490 individuals," *AJR Am J Roentgenol* 2003; 181: 743–8

Schriner, S. E., Linford, N. J., Martin, G. M., et al., "Extension of murine life span by overexpression of catalase targeted to mitochondria," *Science* 2005; 308: 1909–11.

Stathakos, D., Pratsinis, H., Zachos, I., et al., "Greek centenarians: assessment of functional health status and life-style characteristics," *Exp Gerontol* 2005; 40: 512–8.

Terry, D. F., Wilcox, M., McCormick, M. A., Lawler, E., Perls, T. T., "Cardiovascular advantages among the offspring of centenarians," *J Gerontol A Biol Sci Med Sci* 2003; 58: M425–31.

Trichopoulou, A., Costacou, T., Bamia, C., Trichopoulos, D., "Adherence to a Mediterranean diet and survival in a Greek population," *N Engl J Med* 2003; 348: 2599–608.

Vliegenthart, R., Oei, H. H., van den Elzen, A. P., et al., "Alcohol consumption and coronary calcification in a general population," *Arch Intern Med* 2004; 164: 2355–60.

Chapter 7: The Hunt for Procyanidin-Rich Wines

Bergqvist, J., Dokoozlian, N., Ebisuda, N., "Sunlight exposure and temperature effects on berry growth and composition of Cabernet Sauvignon and Grenache in the Central San Joaquin Valley of California," *Am J Enol Vitic* 2001; 52: 1–7.

Cantos, E., Espin, J. C., Fernandez, M. J., Oliva, J., Tomas-Barberan, F. A., "Postharvest UV-C-irradiated grapes as a potential source for producing stilbene-enriched red wines," *J Agric Food Chem* 2003; 51: 1208–14.

Christie, J. M., Jenkins, G.I., "Distinct UV-B and UV-A/blue light signal transduction pathways induce chalcone synthase gene expression in Arabidopsis cells," *Plant Cell* 1996; 8: 1555–67.

Fuleki, T., Ricardo-Da-Silva, J. M., "Effects of cultivar and processing method on the contents of catechins and procyanidins in grape juice," *J Agric Food Chem* 2003; 51: 640–6.

Gollop, R., Even, S., Colova-Tsolova, V., Perl, A., "Expression of the grape dihydroflavonol reductase gene and analysis of its promoter region," *J Exp Bot* 2002; 53: 1397–409.

Gomez-Plaza, E., Gil-Munoz, R., Lopez-Roca, J. M., Martinez, A., "Color and phenolic compounds of a young red wine. Influence of wine-making techniques, storage temperature, and length of storage time," *J Agric Food Chem* 2000; 48: 736–41.

Gonzalez-Manzano, S., Santos-Buelga, C., Perez-Alonso, J. J., Rivas-Gonzalo, J. C., Escribano-Bailon, M. T., "Characterization of the mean degree of polymerization of proanthocyanidins in red wines using liquid chromatography-mass spectrometry (LC-MS)," *J Agric Food Chem* 2006; 54: 4326–32.

Kennedy, J. A., Matthews, M. A., Waterhouse, A. L., "Changes in grape seed polyphenols during fruit ripening," *Phytochemistry* 2000; 55: 77–85.

Lesschaeve, I., Noble, A. C., "Polyphenols: factors influencing their sensory properties and their effects on food and beverage preferences," *Am J Clin Nutr* 2005; 81 (1 Suppl): 330S–5S.

Lindemann, B., "Receptors and transduction in taste," *Nature* 2001; 413: 219–25.

Llaudy, M. C., Canals, R., Canals, J. M., et al., "New method for evaluating astringency in red wine," *J Agric Food Chem* 2004; 52: 742–6.

Monagas, M., Gomez-Cordoves, C., Bartolome, B., Laureano, O., Ricardo da Silva, J. M., "Monomeric, oligomeric, and polymeric flavan-3-ol composition of wines and grapes from Vitis vinifera L. Cv. Graciano, Tempranillo, and Cabernet Sauvignon," *J Agric Food Chem* 2003; 51: 6475–81.

Spayd, S. E., Tarara, J. M., Mee, D. L., Ferguson, J. C., "Separation of Sunlight and Temperature Effects on the Composition of Vitis vinifera cv. Merlot Berries," *Am J Enol Vitic* 2002; 53: 171–82.

CHAPTER 8: MODERATION IS THE MESSAGE

Becker, U., Gronbaek, M., Johansen, D., Sorensen, T. I., "Lower risk for alcohol-induced cirrhosis in wine drinkers," *Hepatology* 2002; 35: 868-75.

Health Claims and Other Health-Related Statements in the Labeling and Advertising of Alcohol Beverages (99R–199P); Final Rule. 27 CFR Parts 4, 5, and 7. Department of Treasury, Alcohol and Tobacco and Trade Bureau, March 3, 2003.

Kamper-Jorgensen, M., Gronbaek, M., Tolstrup, J., Becker, U., "Alcohol and cirrhosis: dose–response or threshold effect?" *J Hepatol* 2004; 41: 25-30.

Klatsky, A. L., Morton, C., Udaltsova, N., Friedman, G. D., "Coffee, cirrhosis, and transaminase enzymes," *Arch Intern Med.* 2006; 166: 1190–5.

Mann, K., Ackermann, K., Croissant, B., et al., "Neuroimaging of gender differences in alcohol dependence: are women more vulnerable?" *Alcohol Clin Exp Res* 2005; 29: 896–901.

Mukamal, K. J., Tolstrup, J. S., Friberg, J., Jensen, G., Gronbaek, M., "Alcohol consumption and risk of atrial fibrillation in men and women: the Copenhagen City Heart Study," *Circulation* 2005; 112: 1736–42.

Pletcher, M. J., Varosy, P., Kiefe, C. I., et al., "Alcohol consumption, binge drinking, and early coronary calcification: findings from the Coronary Artery Risk Development in Young Adults (CARDIA) Study," *Am J Epidemiol* 2005; 161: 423–33.

Rodgers, A., Ezzati, M., Vander Hoorn, S., et al., "Comparative Risk Assessment Collaborating Group. Distribution of major health risks: findings from the Global Burden of Disease study," *PLoS Med* 2004; 1: e27.

Stranges, S., Freudenheim, J. L., Muti, P., et al., "Differential effects of alcohol drinking pattern on liver enzymes in men and women," *Alcohol Clin Exp Res* 2004; 28: 949–56.

Stranges, S., Wu, T., Dorn, J. M., et al., "Relationship of alcohol drinking pattern to risk of hypertension: a population-based study," *Hypertension* 2004; 44: 813–9.

Trevisan, M., Dorn, J., Falkner, K., et al., "Drinking pattern and risk of non-fatal myocardial infarction: a population-based case-control study," *Addiction* 2004; 99: 313–22.

Trevisan, M., Krogh, V., Farinaro, E., Panico, S., Mancini, M., "Alcohol consumption, drinking pattern and blood pressure: analysis of data from the Italian National Research Council Study," *Int J Epidemiol* 1987; 16: 520–7.

Trevisan, M., Schisterman, E., Mennotti, A., Farchi, G., Conti, S., Risk Factor And Life Expectancy Research Group, "Drinking pattern and mortality: the Italian Risk Factor and Life Expectancy pooling project," *Ann Epidemiol* 2001; 11: 312–9.

Walsh, C. R., Larson, M. G., Evans, J. C., et al., "Alcohol consumption and risk for congestive heart failure in the Framingham Heart Study," *Ann Intern Med* 2002; 136: 181–91.

Chapter 9: Seven Diet Myths That Put Your Health at Risk

Abbasi, F., McLaughlin, T., Lamendola, C., et al., "High carbohydrate diets, triglyceride-rich lipoproteins, and coronary heart disease risk," *Am J Cardiol* 2000; 85: 45–8.

Almond, C. S., Shin, A. Y., Fortescue, E. B., et al., "Hyponatremia among runners in the Boston Marathon," *N Engl J Med* 2005; 352: 1550–6.

Bos, M. J., Koudstaal, P. J., Hofman, A., Witteman, J. C., Breteler, M. M., "Uric acid is a risk factor for myocardial infarction and stroke: the Rotterdam study," *Stroke* 2006; 37: 1503–7.

Bray, G. A., Nielsen, S. J., Popkin, B. M., "Consumption of high-fructose corn syrup in beverages may play a role in the epidemic of obesity," *Am J Clin Nutr* 2004; 79: 537–43.

Chao, A., Thun, M. J., Connell, C. J., et al., "Meat consumption and risk of colorectal cancer," *JAMA* 2005; 293: 172–82.

Charest, A., Desroches, S., Vanstone, C. A., Jones, P. J., Lamarche, B., "Unesterified plant sterols and stanols do not affect LDL electrophoretic characteristics in hypercholesterolemic subjects," *J Nutr* 2004; 134: 592–5.

Choi, H. K., Mount, D. B., Reginato, A. M.; American College of Physicians; American Physiological Society, "Pathogenesis of gout," *Ann Intern Med* 2005; 143: 499–516.

Diet, Nutrition and the Prevention of Chronic Diseases. Report of a Joint Expert Consultation for the World Health Organization and the Food and Agriculture Organization of the United Nations. WHO Technical Report Series 916.

Elias, P. K., Elias, M. F., D'Agostino, R. B., Sullivan, L. M., Wolf, P. A., "Serum cholesterol and cognitive performance in the Framingham Heart Study," *Psychosom Med* 2005; 67: 24–30.

German, J. B., Dillard, C. J., "Saturated fats: what dietary intake?" *Am J Clin Nutr* 2004; 80: 550–9.

Global Strategy on Diet, Physical Activity and Health. World Health Organization 2004.

Hooper, L., Summerbell, C.D., Higgins, J.P., et al., "Dietary fat intake and prevention of cardiovascular disease: systematic review," *BMJ* 2001; 322: 757–63.

Miettinen, T. A., Railo, M., Lepantalo, M., Gylling, H., "Plant sterols in serum and in atherosclerotic plaques of patients undergoing carotid endarterectomy," *J Am Coll Cardiol* 2005; 45: 1794–801.

Miyashita, Y., Koide, N., Ohtsuka, M., et al., "Beneficial effect of low carbohydrate in low calorie diets on visceral fat reduction in type 2 diabetic patients with obesity," *Diabetes Res Clin Pract* 2004; 65: 235–41.

Mozaffarian, D., Ascherio, A., Hu, F. B., et al., "Interplay between different polyunsaturated fatty acids and risk of coronary heart disease in men," *Circulation* 2005; 111: 157–64.

Mozaffarian, D., Katan, M. B., Ascherio, A., Stampfer, M. J., Willett, W. C., "Trans fatty acids and cardiovascular disease," *N Engl J Med* 2006; 354: 1601–13.

O'Donovan, D., Feinle-Bisset, C., Wishart, J., Horowitz, M., "Lipase inhibition attenuates the acute inhibitory effects of oral fat on food intake in healthy subjects," *Br J Nutr* 2003; 90: 849–52.

Parks, E. J., Hellerstein, M. K., "Carbohydrate-induced hypertriacylglycerolemia: historical perspective and review of biological mechanisms," *Am J Clin Nutr* 2000; 71: 412–33.

Park, Y., Hunter, D. J., Spiegelman, D., et al., "Dietary fiber intake and risk of colorectal cancer: a pooled analysis of prospective cohort studies," *JAMA* 2005; 294: 2849–57.

Pelkman, C. L., Fishell, V. K., Maddox, D. H., et al., "Effects of moderate-fat (from monounsaturated fat) and low-fat weight-loss diets on the serum lipid profile in overweight and obese men and women," *Am J Clin Nutr* 2004; 79: 204–12.

Salem, J. E., Saidel, G. M., Stanley, W. C., Cabrera, M. E., "Mechanistic model of myocardial energy metabolism under normal and ischemic conditions," *Ann Biomed Eng* 2002; 30: 202–16.

Sehayek, E., Breslow, J. L., "Plasma plant sterol levels: another coronary heart disease risk factor?" *Arterioscler Thromb Vasc Biol* 2005; 25: 5–6.

van Dam, R. M., Hu, F. B., "Coffee consumption and risk of type 2 diabetes: a systematic review," *JAMA* 2005; 294: 97–104.

Wasan, H. S., Goodlad, R.A., "Fibre-supplemented foods may damage your health," *Lancet* 1996; 348: 319–20.

CHAPTER 10: SECRETS FOR PRESERVING A HEALTHY MIND AND BODY

Abbott, R. D., White, L. R., Ross, G. W., et al., "Walking and dementia in physically capable elderly men," *JAMA* 2004; 292: 1447–53.

Appel, L. J., Sacks, F. M., Carey, V. J., et al., "Effects of protein, monounsaturated fat, and carbohydrate intake on blood pressure and serum lipids: results of the OmniHeart randomized trial," *JAMA* 2005; 294: 2455–64.

Arad, Y., Spadaro, L. A., Roth, M., Newstein, D., Guerci, A. D., "Treatment of asymptomatic adults with elevated coronary calcium scores with atorvastatin, vitamin C, and vitamin E: the St. Francis Heart Study randomized clinical trial," *J Am Coll Cardiol* 2005; 46: 166–72.

Ard, J. D., Grambow, S. C., Liu, D., et al., "The effect of the PREMIER interventions on insulin sensitivity," *Diabetes Care* 2004; 27: 340–7.

Barzi, F., Woodward, M., Marfisi, R. M., et al., "Mediterranean diet and all-causes mortality after myocardial infarction: results from the GISSI-Prevenzione trial," *Eur J Clin Nutr* 2003; 57: 604–11.

Baudoin, C., Cohen-Solal, M. E., Beaudreuil, J., De Vernejoul, M. C., "Genetic and environmental factors affect bone density variances of families of men and women with osteoporosis," *J Clin Endocrinol Metab* 2002; 87: 2053–9.

Booth, S. L., Broe, K. E., Gagnon, D. R., et al., "Vitamin K intake and bone mineral density in women and men," *Am J Clin Nutr* 2003; 77: 512–6.

Booth, S. L., Broe, K. E., Peterson, J. W., et al., "Associations between vitamin K biochemical measures and bone mineral density in men and women," *J Clin Endocrinol Metab* 2004; 89: 4904–9.

Bonaa, K. H., Njolstad, I., Ueland, P. M., et al., "Homocysteine lowering and cardiovascular events after acute myocardial infarction," *N Engl J Med* 2006; 354: 1578–88.

Cho, E., Seddon, J. M., Rosner, B., Willett, W. C., Hankinson, S.E., "Prospective study of intake of fruits, vegetables, vitamins, and carotenoids and risk of age-related maculopathy," *Arch Ophthalmol* 2004; 122: 883–92.

Desvarieux, M., Demmer, R. T., Rundek, T., et al., "Periodontal microbiota and carotid intima-media thickness: the Oral Infections and Vascular Disease Epidemiology Study (INVEST)," *Circulation* 2005; 111: 576–82.

Diwadkar-Navsariwala, V., Diamond, A.M., "The link between selenium and chemoprevention: a case for selenoproteins," *J Nutr* 2004; 134: 2899-902.

Elliott, P., Stamler, J., Dyer, A. R., et al., "Association between protein intake and blood pressure: the INTERMAP Study," *Arch Intern Med* 2006; 166: 79–87.

Food, Nutrition and the Prevention of Cancer: a global perspective. World Cancer Research Fund/American Institute for Cancer Research. 1997.

Giannopoulou, I., Ploutz-Snyder, L. L., Carhart, R., et al., "Exercise is required for visceral fat loss in postmenopausal women with type 2 diabetes." *J Clin Endocrinol Metab* 2005; 90: 1511–8.

Gill, J. M., Al-Mamari, A., Ferrell, W. R., et al., "Effects of prior moderate exercise on postprandial metabolism and vascular function in lean and centrally obese men," *J Am Coll Cardiol* 2004; 44: 2375–82.

Gill, J.M., Al-Mamari, A., Ferrell, W. R., et al., "Effects of a moderate exercise session on postprandial lipoproteins, apolipoproteins and lipoprotein remnants in middle-aged men," *Atherosclerosis* 2006; 185: 87–96.

Gonzalez-Ortiz, M., Martinez-Abundis, E., Balcazar-Munoz, B. R., Pascoe-Gonzalez, S., "Effect of sleep deprivation on insulin sensitivity and cortisol concentration in healthy subjects," *Diabetes Nutr Metab* 2000; 13: 80–3.

Gottlieb, D.J., Punjabi, N. M., Newman, A. B., et al., "Association of sleep time with diabetes mellitus and impaired glucose tolerance," *Arch Intern Med* 2005; 165: 863–7.

He, J., Gu, D., Wu, X., et al., "Effect of soybean protein on blood pressure: a randomized, controlled trial," *Ann Intern Med* 2005; 143: 1–9.

Hercberg, S., "The history of beta-carotene and cancers: from observational to intervention studies. What lessons can be drawn for future research on polyphenols?" *Am J Clin Nutr* 2005; 81 (1 Suppl): 218S–222S.

Hercberg, S., Galan, P., Preziosi, P., et al., "The SU.VI.MAX Study: a randomized, placebo-controlled trial of the health effects of antioxidant vitamins and minerals," *Arch Intern Med* 2004; 164: 2335–42.

Holick, M. F., "Vitamin D: importance in the prevention of cancers, type 1 diabetes, heart disease, and osteoporosis," *Am J Clin Nutr* 2004; 79: 362–71.

Iestra, J. A., Kromhout, D., van der Schouw, Y. T., et al., "Effect size estimates of lifestyle and dietary changes on all-cause mortality in coronary artery disease patients: a systematic review," *Circulation* 2005; 112: 924–34.

Ilich, J. Z., Brownbill, R. A., Tamborini, L., Crncevic-Orlic, Z., "To drink or not to drink: how are alcohol, caffeine and past smoking related to bone mineral density in elderly women?" *J Am Coll Nutr* 2002; 21: 536–44.

John, J. H., Ziebland, S., Yudkin, P., Roe, L. S., Neil, H. A.; Oxford Fruit and Vegetable Study Group, "Effects of fruit and vegetable consumption on plasma antioxidant concentrations and blood pressure: a randomised controlled trial," *Lancet* 2002; 359: 1969–74.

Kawakami, N., Takatsuka, N., Shimizu, H., "Sleep disturbance and onset of type 2 diabetes," *Diabetes Care* 2004; 27: 282–3.

Khaw, K. T., Bingham, S., Welch, A., et al., "Relation between plasma ascorbic acid and mortality in men and women in EPIC-Norfolk prospective study: a prospective population study, European Prospective Investigation into Cancer and Nutrition," *Lancet* 2001; 357: 657–63.

Khaw, K. T., Jakes, R., Bingham, S., et al., "Work and leisure time physical activity assessed using a simple, pragmatic, validated questionnaire and incident cardiovascular disease and all-cause mortality in men and women: The European Prospective Investigation into Cancer in Norfolk prospective population study," *Int J Epidemiol* 2006; 35: 1034–43.

Knoops, K. T., de Groot, L. C., Kromhout, D., et al.,"Mediterranean diet, lifestyle factors, and 10-year mortality in elderly European men and women: the HALE project," *JAMA* 2004; 292: 1433–9.

Marchioli, R., Levantesi, G., Macchia, A., et al., "Vitamin E increases the risk of developing heart failure after myocardial infarction: results from the GISSI-Prevenzione trial." *J Cardiovasc Med* (Hagerstown) 2006; 7: 347-50.

Mares-Perlman, J. A., Millen, A. E., Ficek, T. L., Hankinson, S. E., "The body of evidence to support a protective role for lutein and zeaxanthin in delaying chronic disease. Overview," *J Nutr* 2002; 132: 518S–524S.

McCabe, L. D., Martin, B. R., McCabe, G. P., et al., "Dairy intakes affect bone density in the elderly," *Am J Clin Nutr* 2004; 80: 1066–74.

Moat, S. J., Doshi, S. N., Lang, D., et al., "Treatment of coronary heart disease with folic acid: is there a future?" *Am J Physiol* 2004; 287: H1–7.

Miller, E. R. 3rd, Pastor-Barriuso, R., Dalal, D., et al., "Meta-analysis: high-dosage vitamin E supplementation may increase all-cause mortality," *Ann Intern Med* 2005; 142: 37–46.

Mosekilde, L., "Vitamin D and the elderly," *Clin Endocrinol* (Oxf) 2005; 62: 265–81.

Nieves, J. W., "Osteoporosis: the role of micronutrients," *Am J Clin Nutr* 2005; 81: 1232S–9S.

Qualified Health Claims: Letter of Enforcement Discretion—Walnuts and Coronary Heart Disease. U.S. Food and Drug Administration. March 9, 2004.

Renaud, S., de Lorgeril, M., Delaye, J., et al., "Cretan Mediterranean diet for prevention of coronary heart disease," *Am J Clin Nutr* 1995; 61 (6 Suppl): 1360S–7S.

Roberts, C. K., Barnard, R. J., "Effects of exercise and diet on chronic disease," *J Appl Physiol* 2005; 98: 3–30

Rozanski, A., Blumenthal, J. A., Davidson, K. W., Saab, P. G., Kubzansky, L., "The epidemiology, pathophysiology, and management of psychosocial risk factors in cardiac practice: the emerging field of behavioral cardiology," *J Am Coll Cardiol* 2005; 45: 637–51.

Rumsfeld, J. S., Ho, P. M., "Depression and cardiovascular disease: a call for recognition," *Circulation* 2005; 111: 250–3.

Sacks, F. M., Svetkey, L. P., Vollmer, W. M., et al., "Effects on blood pressure of reduced dietary sodium and the Dietary Approaches to Stop Hypertension (DASH) diet," DASH-Sodium Collaborative Research Group, *N Engl J Med* 2001; 344: 3–10.

Simopoulos, A.P., "The Mediterranean diets: What is so special about the diet of Greece? The scientific evidence," *J Nutr* 2001; 131 (11 Suppl): 3065S–73S.

Spiegel, K., Tasali, E., Penev, P., Van Cauter, E., "Brief communication: Sleep curtailment in healthy young men is associated with decreased leptin levels, elevated ghrelin levels, and increased hunger and appetite," *Ann Intern Med* 2004; 141: 846–50.

Stamler, J., Elliott, P., Appel, L., et al., "Higher blood pressure in middle-aged American adults with less education—role of multiple dietary factors: the INTERMAP study," *J Hum Hypertens* 2003; 17: 655–775.

Tapsell, L. C., Gillen, L. J., Patch, C. S., et al., "Including walnuts in a low-fat/modified-fat diet improves HDL cholesterol-to-total cholesterol ratios in patients with type 2 diabetes," *Diabetes Care* 2004; 27: 2777–83.

Taylor, P. R., Parnes, H. L., Lippman, S. M., "Science peels the onion of selenium effects on prostate carcinogenesis," *J Natl Cancer Inst* 2004; 96: 645–7.

Tseng, M., Breslow, R. A., Graubard, B. I., Ziegler, R. G., "Dairy, calcium, and vitamin D intakes and prostate cancer risk in the National Health and Nutrition Examination Epidemiologic Follow-up Study cohort," *Am J Clin Nutr* 2005; 81: 1147–54.

van Gelder, B. M., Tijhuis, M. A., Kalmijn, S., et al., "Physical activity in relation to cognitive decline in elderly men: the FINE Study," *Neurology* 2004; 63: 2316–21.

Wang, J. S., Li, Y. S., Chen, J. C., Chen, Y. W., "Effects of exercise training and deconditioning on platelet aggregation induced by alternating shear stress in men," *Arterioscler Thromb Vasc Biol* 2005; 25: 454–60.

Weigle, D. S., Breen, P. A., Matthys, C. C., et al., "A high-protein diet induces sustained reductions in appetite, ad libitum caloric intake, and body weight despite compensatory changes in diurnal plasma leptin and ghrelin concentrations," *Am J Clin Nutr* 2005; 82: 41–8.

Weuve, J., Kang, J. H., Manson, J. E., et al., "Physical activity, including walking, and cognitive function in older women," *JAMA* 2004; 292: 1454–61.

Zambon, D., Sabate, J., Munoz, S., et al., "Substituting walnuts for monounsaturated fat improves the serum lipid profile of hypercholesterolemic men and women. A randomized crossover trial," *Ann Intern Med* 2000; 132: 538–46.

Zureik, M., Galan, P., Bertrais, S., et al., "Effects of long-term daily low-dose supplementation with antioxidant vitamins and minerals on structure and function of large arteries," *Arterioscler Thromb Vasc Biol* 2004; 24: 1485–91.

Chapter 11: A Guide to Complete Nutrition

Adolfsson, O., Meydani, S. N., Russell, R. M., "Yogurt and gut function," *Am J Clin Nutr* 2004; 80: 245–56.

Brenner, H., Rothenbacher, D., Bode, G., Adler, G., "Inverse graded relation between alcohol consumption and active infection with Helicobacter pylori," *Am J Epidemiol* 1999; 149: 571–6.

Brouwer, I. A., Heeringa, J., Geleijnse, J. M., Zock, P. L., Witteman, J. C., "Intake of very long-chain n–3 fatty acids from fish and incidence of atrial fibrillation. The Rotterdam Study," *Am Heart J* 2006; 151: 857–62.

Carmel, R., "Prevalence of undiagnosed pernicious anemia in the elderly," *Arch Intern Med* 1996; 156: 1097–100.

Djousse, L., Arnett, D. K., Carr, J. J., et al., "Dietary linolenic acid is inversely associated with calcified atherosclerotic plaque in the coronary arteries: the National Heart, Lung, and Blood Institute Family Heart Study," *Circulation* 2005; 111: 2921–6.

Franco, O. H., Bonneux, L., de Laet, C., et al., "The Polymeal: a more natural, safer, and probably tastier (than the Polypill) strategy to reduce cardiovascular disease by more than 75%," *BMJ* 2004; 329: 1447–50.

Frost, L., Vestergaard, P., "n–3 Fatty acids consumed from fish and risk of atrial fibrillation or flutter: the Danish Diet, Cancer, and Health Study," *Am J Clin Nutr* 2005; 81: 50–4.

Hampl, J. S., Taylor, C. A., Johnston, C. S., "Vitamin C deficiency and depletion in the United States: the Third National Health and Nutrition Examination Survey, 1988 to 1994," *Am J Public Health* 2004; 94: 870–5.

He, F. J., Nowson, C. A., MacGregor, G. A., "Fruit and vegetable consumption and stroke: meta-analysis of cohort studies," *Lancet* 2006; 367: 320–6.

He, K., Liu, K., Daviglus, M. L., Morris, S. J., et al., "Magnesium intake and incidence of metabolic syndrome among young adults," *Circulation* 2006; 113: 1675–82.

Human Vitamin and Mineral Requirements. Report of a joint FAO/WHO expert consultation 2001.

Koh-Banerjee, P., Franz, M., Sampson, L., et al., "Changes in whole-grain, bran, and cereal fiber consumption in relation to 8-y weight gain among men," *Am J Clin Nutr* 2004; 80: 1237–45.

Laaksonen, D. E., Niskanen, L., Nyyssonen, K., et al., "C-reactive protein in the prediction of cardiovascular and overall mortality in middle-aged men: a population-based cohort study," *Eur Heart J* 2005; 26: 1783–9.

Montonen, J., Jarvinen, R., Heliovaara, M., et al., "Food consumption and the incidence of type II diabetes mellitus," *Eur J Clin Nutr* 2005; 59: 441–8.

Morris, M. C., Evans, D. A., Tangney, C. C., Bienias, J. L., Wilson, R. S., "Fish consumption and cognitive decline with age in a large community study," *Arch Neurol* 2005; 62: 1849–53.

Mozaffarian, D., Psaty, B. M., Rimm, E. B., et al., "Fish intake and risk of incident atrial fibrillation," *Circulation* 2004 27; 110: 368–73.

Qualified Health Claims: Monounsaturated Fatty Acids from Olive Oil and Coronary Heart Disease (Docket No 2003Q–0559). U.S. Food and Drug Administration. Nov. 1, 2004.

Raitt, M. H, Connor, W. E., Morris, C., et al., "Fish oil supplementation and risk of ventricular tachycardia and ventricular fibrillation in patients with implantable defibrillators: a randomized controlled trial," *JAMA* 2005; 293: 2884–91.

Rowland, I. R., Wiseman, H., Sanders, T. A., Adlercreutz, H., Bowey, E. A., "Interindividual variation in metabolism of soy isoflavones and lignans: influence of habitual diet on equol production by the gut microflora," *Nutr Cancer* 2000; 36: 27–32

Sacks, F. M., "Dietary phytoestrogens to prevent cardiovascular disease: early promise unfulfilled," *Circulation* 2005; 111: 385–7.

Schulman, S. P., Becker, L. C., Kass, D. A., et al., "L-arginine therapy in acute myocardial infarction: the Vascular Interaction With Age in Myocardial Infarction (VINTAGE MI) randomized clinical trial," *JAMA* 2006; 295: 58–64.

Setchell, K. D., Clerici, C., Lephart, E. D., et al., "S-equol, a potent ligand for estrogen receptor beta, is the exclusive enantiomeric form of the soy isoflavone metabolite produced by human intestinal bacterial flora," *Am J Clin Nutr* 2005; 81: 1072–9.

Siscovick, D. S., Raghunathan, T., King, I., et al., "Dietary intake of long-chain n–3 polyunsaturated fatty acids and the risk of primary cardiac arrest," *Am J Clin Nutr* 2000; 71 (1 Suppl): 208S–12S.

U.S. Food and Information Center: Dietary Reference Intakes (DRI) and Recommended Dietary Allowances (RDA).

van der Schouw, Y. T., Kreijkamp-Kaspers, S., Peeters, P. H., et al., "Prospective study on usual dietary phytoestrogen intake and cardiovascular disease risk in Western women," *Circulation* 2005; 111: 465–71.

Virtanen, J. K., Voutilainen, S., Rissanen, T. H., et al., "High dietary methionine intake increases the risk of acute coronary events in middle-aged men," *Nutr Metab Cardiovasc Dis* 2006; 16: 113–20.

Virtanen, J. K., Voutilainen, S., Rissanen, T. H., et al., "Mercury, fish oils, and risk of acute coronary events and cardiovascular disease, coronary heart disease, and all-cause mortality in men in eastern Finland," *Arterioscler Thromb Vasc Biol* 2005; 25: 228–33.

Willett, W. C., Sacks, F., Trichopoulou, A., et al., "Mediterranean diet pyramid: a cultural model for healthy eating," *Am J Clin Nutr* 1995; 61 (6 Suppl): 1402S–6S.

Wolters, M., Strohle, A., Hahn, A., "Cobalamin: a critical vitamin in the elderly," *Prev Med* 2004; 39: 1256–66.

Zampelas, A., Panagiotakos, D. B., Pitsavos, C., et al., "Fish consumption among healthy adults is associated with decreased levels of inflammatory markers related to cardiovascular disease: the ATTICA study," *J Am Coll Cardiol* 2005; 46: 120–4.

Zhang, X., Shu, X. O., Li, H., et al., "Prospective cohort study of soy food consumption and risk of bone fracture among postmenopausal women," *Arch Intern Med* 2005; 165: 1890–5.

GLOSSARY

Advanced Glycation End Products (AGEs) These are formed by spontaneous chemical reactions of glucose, particularly with proteins, which lead to damaged proteins that no longer function normally and can trigger vascular disease. AGEs are a particular problem in cases of poorly controlled diabetes.

Alpha-linoleic acid An 18-carbon polyunsaturated omega-6 essential fatty acid, which is abundant in seeds, nuts, and vegetable oils. It is a precursor to arachidonic acid. Excess consumption is thought to contribute to an imbalance with omega-3 fatty acids and promote inflammation.

Alpha-linolenic acid (ALA) An 18-carbon polyunsaturated omega-3 essential fatty acid, present in plant sources such as flaxseed, hemp seed, walnuts, and dark green leafy vegetables. It can be a precursor for synthesis of longer omega-3 PUFAs EPA and DHA.

Amino acid The building block of proteins. Proteins are composed of twenty different amino acids. Eight of these are referred to as essential amino acids because they cannot be made in the body and we rely on dietary sources to stay healthy. See Chapter 11.

Angina (pectoris) Chest pain due to lack of adequate blood supply to the heart muscle. Generally caused by obstruction of the coronary arteries by atherosclerosis. Often triggered by exercise and disappears at rest.

Anthocyanins Red, purple, and blue pigments in some vegetables (red cabbage and red onions), and fruits such as berries, cherries, and red grapes—and therefore red wine; a type of flavonoid.

Antioxidant   Any substance that delays or stops oxidation reactions.

Arachidonic acid   A 20-carbon omega-6 fatty acid occurring in animal cells; a metabolic precursor of several groups of biologically active substances, including prostaglandins.

Arginine   An amino acid that helps to maintain a healthy vascular system by acting within blood vessel walls to keep them relaxed and promote blood flow.

Arteriosclerosis   The loss of elasticity and thickening of the walls of the arteries that generally occurs with increasing age.

Artery   A muscular blood vessel forming part of the circulation system; usually carrying oxygen-rich blood from the heart.

Atherosclerosis   A form of arteriosclerosis characterized by the degeneration of the arteries because of the buildup of fatty deposits called atheromatous plaques.

Basal metabolic rate (BMR)   The speed at which one's body burns calories while resting.

Beta-carotene   A carotenoid that can act as a precursor for vitamin A synthesis. It also has antioxidant properties.

Betacyanins   Red to purple pigments such as betanin in beets—structurally unrelated to anthocyanins.

Body mass index (BMI)   A measure of body fat based on height and weight. See page 277 for how to calculate your BMI.

Carbohydrates   Molecules composed of sugars. Simple carbohydrates are individual sugar molecules such as glucose or fructose, or two sugars bonded together such as sucrose (table sugar). Complex carbohydrates are long chains of sugars; they are used for storage in plants. Simple carbohydrates are rapidly absorbed, but complex carbohydrates need to be digested before absorption occurs. Some complex plant carbohydrates cannot be digested; these are known as dietary fiber.

Cardiovascular disease (CVD)   A general term for diseases of the heart and blood vessels (arteries or veins).

Carotene, carotenoids   Red, orange, and yellow pigments found in the leaves and fruits of many plants, which act as precursors to vitamin A and as antioxidants.

Catechin and epicatechin   Flavanols found in cocoa, grapes, red wine, green tea, black tea.

Cell membrane   The wall that surrounds each living cell of all organisms; it is made up of proteins and fats (phospholipids).

Cholesterol   A fatty substance (lipid) found in the cell membranes of all body tissues, including the blood. It is produced by the body and also supplied by the food we eat. High levels in the blood contribute to atherosclerosis.

Coenzyme Q$_{10}$ A fat-soluble, vitaminlike molecule that plays a key role in energy production in all cells.

Coronary heart disease (CHD) or coronary artery disease   A term to describe atherosclerosis in the coronary arteries, which can cause angina and lead to myocardial infarction (heart attack) and sudden death.

Degenerative disease   Progressive deterioration of function of tissues or organs over time.

Diabetes mellitus   A disorder characterized by a deficiency in insulin, leading to problems in the regulation of blood sugar (glucose) levels, which in turn leads to severe health problems through the harmful effects of constantly high glucose levels.

Diuretic   An agent that increases the flow of urine.

Docosahexaenoic acid (DHA) An important long-chain 22-carbon omega-3 fatty acid that helps protect from heart disease and plays a key role in optimal brain function. Many diets are deficient in DHA. It is present in large amounts in oily fish such as herring, mackerel, salmon, sardines, and tuna, and to a lesser extent in meat from grass-fed animals. Omega-3-enriched eggs from chicken fed a vegetarian diet including algal extracts as a natural source of DHA are another good source. May be produced in small amounts from dietary alpha-linolenic acid.

Eicosapentaenoic acid (EPA) A 20-carbon omega-3 fatty acid that is a precursor in the synthesis of DHA. It can be converted to prostaglandins with less inflammatory activity. Food sources are the same as DHA.

Ellagic acid A polyphenol acid that reacts with glucose to form ellagitannins. Present in raspberries, pomegranates, and walnuts.

Endothelin-1 A 21-amino-acid peptide produced by the endothelium with vasoconstrictor actions and an important role in maintaining the structure of artery walls. In excess it contributes to the development of atherosclerosis.

Endothelium A single layer of cells lining the blood vessels, heart, and lymphatic vessels.

Enzymes Complex proteins that are produced by living cells and act as catalysts in specific biochemical reactions.

Epicatechin See Catechin.

Epidemiology The study of the incidence and distribution of diseases and of other factors relating to health across populations.

Essential fatty acid (EFA) Omega-3 and omega-6 are fatty acids that are essential to life but cannot be made by the body and must be obtained from food. Sources include oily fish, nuts, flaxseed, vegetable oils, and dark green vegetables.

Fatty acids Consist of a chain of carbon atoms with an acidic group at one end. The carbon chain is described as saturated or unsaturated depending on the presence of carbon atoms that have the maximum of hydrogen atoms (saturated) or have double bonds (unsaturated) that could react with further hydrogen. *Monounsaturated* refers to fatty acids with a single double bond; *polyunsaturated* refers to fatty acids with several double bonds.

Fiber A term for the carbohydrate components of plants—fruits, vegetables, nuts, and whole grains—that cannot be digested. They nonetheless play a vital part in the process of digestion and bowel function. Vegetables, fruits, pulses, and whole-grain cereals and breads are good sources. There are two types of fiber: insoluble, which does not dissolve in water, and soluble, which will dissolve in water and can be partially or completely broken down by bacteria in the large intestine to provide a source of nutrients with health properties. Soluble fiber helps to stabilize blood sugar and may reduce blood cholesterol (particularly LDL cholesterol), thus reducing the risk of heart disease; oats, beans, apples, and citrus fruits are good sources.

Fining An agent used to clarify wine because of its ability to bind and precipitate particulate components.

Flavanol A specific type of flavonoid.

Flavonoid A group of polyphenol phytochemicals that are abundant in fruits, flowers, cocoa, and some nuts.

Free radical An unstable molecule containing at least one unpaired electron, which interacts with other molecules and causes oxidation. Oxidation causes cell damage, resulting in disease and premature aging.

Gene A unit of heredity composed of DNA occupying a fixed position on a chromosome.

Glucose A simple sugar that is the main source of energy in many cellular processes.

Glycemic index (GI)   An index of the readily absorbable sugars present in food. The higher the rate of absorption of sugars into the blood, the higher the glycemic index.

Glycemic load (GL)   An index of the total digestible sugar in a given portion of food.

High density lipoprotein (HDL)   Lipoproteins that carry cholesterol to the liver for breakdown and excretion from the body. Also known as "good cholesterol."

Homocysteine   A metabolic breakdown product of methionine, an essential amino acid found in protein. High levels of homocysteine can increase the risk of heart disease, memory loss, and Alzheimer's disease.

Hypoglycemia   Low blood sugar (glucose).

Insulin   A protein hormone, secreted by the pancreas, that controls the concentration of glucose in the blood.

Insulin resistance   Loss of sensitivity to insulin in muscle, fat, and liver, resulting in slow uptake of glucose from blood.

Ischemia   A reduction of the blood supply to a tissue or organ of the body.

Ischemic stroke   A stroke resulting from an insufficient supply of blood to the brain, or part of the brain, often resulting from a blood clot caused by atherosclerosis in the neck.

Lipid   A general term for fatty substances, including fatty acids, triglycerides, and cholesterol.

Lipoprotein   A protein complex that is a combination of protein and lipid; lipoproteins act as transporters for cholesterol.

Low density lipoprotein (LDL) Lipoproteins that transport cholesterol to body tissues. High LDL-cholesterol can lead to artery damage. Also known as "bad cholesterol."

Lutein A type of carotenoid, which, along with the closely related compound zeaxanthin, plays a key role in macula function in the eye.

Macular degeneration The progressive deterioration in function of the light-sensitive cells of the eye, leading to loss of sight.

Metabolic syndrome A combination of medical symptoms that includes obesity, diabetes or insulin resistance, high blood pressure, low HDL-cholesterol, and raised triglycerides. Also called syndrome X.

Metabolism The sum of all the biochemical processes that occur in living cells. It is also often used to refer to the interplay between nutrient intake, utilization, and energy production.

Microbiology The branch of biology involving the study of microorganisms and their effects on humans.

Micronutrient Any substance, such as a vitamin, mineral, or trace element, essential for healthy growth and development.

Mitochondria Structures responsible for energy production in cells.

Myocardial infarction Commonly referred to as heart attack, caused by the obstruction of a coronary artery by a blood clot, which leads to the death of an area of heart muscle due to starvation of oxygen.

Obesity A condition defined by above-normal body weight, usually with a BMI of 30 or above.

Oleic acid An 18-carbon monounsaturated fatty acid found in almost all plant and animal fats and oils. .

Omega-6 Polyunsaturated fatty acids found in all vegetable oils, seeds, and nuts.

Omega-3 Polyunsaturated fatty acids found in fish and some vegetable sources (see ALA, DHA, and EPA, above).

Osteoporosis A condition in which bone structure is modified and weakened, leading to an increased risk of fractures.

Oxidation The result of a chemical reaction with oxygen. Associated with aging, but is also an important part of the body's defense system to prevent infection.

Oxidative stress Occurs when highly reactive forms of oxygen, sometimes referred to as free radicals, damage proteins and DNA. Prolonged oxidative stress causes damage to cells to accumulate and the cells to either fail to function properly or die.

Paraoxonase An HDL-associated enzyme that helps prevent oxidation of LDL.

Peptide A group of compounds consisting of two or more amino acids.

Phenol Molecules containing one or more hydroxyl groups bound directly to a carbon atom in an atomic ring.

Phytochemical, phytonutrient A chemical substance from a plant source.

Phytosterols Plant chemicals (sterols) that are added to food to block cholesterol absorption and to reduce LDL cholesterol.

Platelet A minute cell-like particle that is critical for normal blood clotting, but may sometimes become too sticky in patients with heart disease, which can increase the risk of blood clots and can cause heart attack or stroke.

Polyphenol Any chemical compound having more than one phenol group.

Polyunsaturated fatty acids (PUFAs)   Omega-3 and omega-6 fatty acids.

Prebiotic   Complex carbohydrates that promote the growth of healthy bacteria in the colon.

Proanthocyanidin   An alternative name for procyanidin.

Probiotic   Dietary supplements and foods containing potentially healthy bacteria, which can improve intestinal function.

Procyanidin   A type of flavonoid consisting mainly of epicatechin and catechin in short chains referred to as oligomers.

Prostacyclin   A biologically active lipid synthesized from arachidonic acid that is a vasodilator and inhibits platelet function to prevent blood clotting.

Prostaglandin   A type of biologically active lipid that plays a key role in inflammation.

Protein   A molecule composed of one or more chains of amino acids. Key structural and biochemical functions of all cells are dependent on their protein constituents.

Pycnogenol   Procyanidins extracted from pine bark.

Statin   A type of medicine that inhibits cholesterol production and helps lower LDL-cholesterol.

Syndrome X   See Metabolic syndrome.

Theobromine   A substance found in cocoa similar in structure to caffeine, which also causes stimulatory effects.

Therapeutics   The branch of medicine concerned with the treatment and cure of disease.

Trans fats   Hydrogenated fats found in solid or semisolid vegetable-oil-based products, such as margarine, and in many baked products and prepared foods. To produce these fats, hydrogen gas is bubbled through vegetable oil in the presence of chemical catalysts. This process changes the chemical structure of the fats to such an extent that the body finds it hard to metabolize them. Trans fats have been linked to an increased risk of numerous diseases, including cancer, diabetes, irregular heartbeat, and atherosclerosis.

Triglycerides   Three fatty acid molecules linked to one glycerol molecule. This is the most common form of natural fat molecules found in food and produced by the body. Triglycerides circulate in the bloodstream, transported by lipoproteins, which also carry cholesterol. As a result, high triglyceride levels can be a sign of high cholesterol. High triglyceride levels are linked to a greater risk of heart disease.

Vascular   Relating to blood vessels.

Vasoconstriction   The constriction of blood vessels resulting in high blood pressure.

Vasodilation   Relaxation and widening of blood vessels, leading to lower blood pressure.

Vein   A blood vessel forming part of the circulation system; usually carrying oxygen-depleted blood to the heart.

Visceral fat   Fat that accumulates in the abdomen around the intestines and other key organs. This type of body fat is associated with an increased risk of developing insulin resistance and diabetes.

acknowledgments

My thanks go to Jancis Robinson and other members of the Geoffrey Roberts Award committee, whose backing encouraged me to delve into the relationship between wine consumption and longevity. Thanks also to Adrian Webster, who convinced me to write this book so that more people could understand the importance of eating well, drinking red wine in moderation, and living a longer, healthier life. I am particularly grateful for the efforts of Maggie Ramsay, whose editorial input during the writing of this book has been immense and invaluable.

Special thanks go to my many colleagues and collaborators who have been involved in this research over the past few years, and without whom I would not have been able to write this book. I am also indebted to the many winemakers and producers who have given me their time and provided wine samples for my laboratory analyses.

315

index